Why we cheat
When we eat
and
How to stop

CLARE TAYLOR

DEDICATION

To everyone who has ever tried to diet and failed, to all those men and women who hate their bodies, to every person who feels hopeless about their weight and powerless over food.
This is for you.

CONTENTS

ACKNOWLEDGMENTS

Particular thanks to Anita Paddock, Rachel Laws and Rebecca
Blackburn for editorial assistance.
Thank you most of all to Tony for your constancy and support.

It takes a thief to catch a thief

There is a saying 'it takes one to know one', and nowhere is that truer than in this book. I could not have written it without being the ultimate cheat when it comes to food and dieting. I have failed at every diet, snuck food in every conceivable way and broken every resolution to lose weight. I know what it's like.

I have also found a way through it, a way to lose the weight, maintain it (for twenty years at this point) and have a healthy body without being obsessed by food or permanently on a restricted eating plan.

In my early twenties I put on a lot of weight. Within three months of leaving university I was suddenly five kilograms heavier. I had secured a fabulous job and was on track to become a senior player in the corporate world, or 'corpulent' world in my case.

My employer was Cadbury and my role was to manage the Crunchie plant, in a chocolate factory. It was a vast Victorian building that oozed chocolate. You could smell its luscious aroma for miles. Large bath tubs of molten chocolate would roll past as I sat in my office. Conveyor belts of confectionary thundered by, day and night, vanishing into the distance. Occasionally, some equipment would malfunction and chocolate bars would shoot onto the floor, to be swept up and fed to the local pigs (lucky swine). You don't need to be a detective to work out the cause of my sudden increase in girth.

I have a small frame and within a year I was ten kilos heavier. Zips gaped or refused to close. Flesh bulged over my waistband and my upper arms took on terrifying proportions. When friends and relatives saw me, they stepped back, did a double-take and tried to hide a look of horror.

The slender student of a year back had vanished beneath a rippling tide.

I felt ashamed. Worse - I felt fat and ashamed. I wanted to lose weight more than anything, more than anything in the world. As a determined and motivated person, I felt sure it couldn't be too hard. I'd already completed a degree and scored a top job. I was fired up (desperate is a better description) and armed with the latest diet.

So why then didn't I succeed? Why didn't the weight drop off?

Time and again, I would cheat. I would sabotage my own attempts to diet. I would sneak food, nibble relentlessly, shove stuff into my mouth when no one was looking. The harder I dieted, the worse I cheated.

The more I cheated, the more I hated myself. And the more I hated myself, the worse I ate and the fatter I got. Ten kilos because fifteen.

Bizarrely enough, my weight problems didn't start in earnest until I started dieting. Or maybe that's true for most of us?

As the weight crept on, my self esteem crept out the door. Occasionally, I felt so obsessed by food that I struggled in social situations. If someone asked about my weekend, all I could think about was what I'd eaten. Sometimes, no, often, I thought I looked too fat to be acceptable. I stopped going on dates, in case anyone put their arm around me and felt my rolls of fat. I stopped hanging out with girlfriends in case they commented on my appearance. And as for the prospect of anyone seeing me naked – well, that was just not on the cards.

I withdrew. I felt increasingly isolated, out of control. I was lonely, miserable. By this time I had put on 15kg (two stone or 25lbs). I hated what I saw in the mirror. I was ugly and worthless.

That seems a long time ago now. It seems like a different person.

It has been a long, slow journey for me. I had to try all the diets – the food combining, low fat, low carb, vegetarian, blood type.... Oh I tried them all. They just made me feel depressed and compulsive. I found myself unhappy and hungry, thinking about all the foods I couldn't have, that I wanted to eat but were forbidden.

My saviour was a notion that is so obvious and so straightforward that it seems unfeasible. To eat when I was hungry, to eat exactly what I was hungry for, and to stop when I was full. Boy was that difficult. Firstly to tell when I was hungry. And then to work out what I actually wanted to eat through all the rules, forbidden foods, portion control and binges. What did I actually like eating? I don't think I even knew.

It took me a long time to work it out. I spent two years not eating salads until I was ready to admit that I enjoyed them again. It was six years until I rediscovered red meat and its rich, tasty delights. It was ten years before I could let go of chocolate enough to have a bar in the house and enjoy it, a square at a time. It took me a decade or so to work it out and lose the weight permanently. But I got there.

I ate a square a chocolate today. From a bar that I've had in my cupboard for a week. I had a square two days ago and I haven't felt like eating any more until today. Amazing huh? I wouldn't have believed that was me. I never believed people who claimed that they could do that. How can you be so, well, so offhand about chocolate? And how can you eat whatever you like and still be thinner than you were when you were dieting?

All the weight is gone now. I never weigh myself. I eat what I like. I have no forbidden foods. I eat chocolate, ice cream, dessert, butter, cream, crisps. And salads, chicken, juicy mangoes, yoghurt. I eat all my favourite foods. I never binge. I never diet. And my weight just looks after itself. It sounds too good to be true. I can hardly believe it is true myself some days.

Twenty five years ago, I wanted to be thin so badly that I was prepared to cut off my left arm (which would certainly have reduced my weight). And yet I was compelled to consistently break my diet and undermine my efforts. Why?

All over the world, sane, successful, intelligent people resolve to go on healthy eating plans, and then find themselves eating the very foods that they've just sworn off. Why?

Why do we cheat when we eat?

The piercing heartbreak and urgency of this question has fuelled a twenty year hunt for the answer. I read science journals, interviewed nutritionists and medics, and scoured the latest research for answers. I've looked into Psychology, Neuroscience, Medicine, Anatomy, Addiction, Social Science, Cultural studies and more. The information I found, helped me shed the weight and keep it off for two decades. It wasn't easy - it's far easier to follow a six point diet plan - but it has worked.

I hope this book can fast track some of those things for you. I had to work out much of it from scratch. I had to put aside the diet books and rhetoric in order to discover something else. As I did so, I began to realise that science already knew what I had worked so hard to uncover. There is hard evidence behind what was working for me. It strikes me as incredible that it isn't more widely known and publicised.

It turns out that there are many reasons why we cheat, none of the them the ones that I had both suspected and feared. When I was struggling with food, I was certain that it must be because I was a bad person, or lazy or weak-willed or deserved to be fat.

Once we understand what's driving our behaviour, we can do things differently, try something new, and stop sabotaging our own efforts. Some people may be more vulnerable to certain triggers, and others may be undermined by different factors. As you read, you will find what resonates with you.

If you want to know why we cheat when we eat, read on. When we know the 'why', we can find solutions.

I did and I hope you can too.

CHAPTER ONE
HOW WE SET OURSELVES UP TO FAIL

In this first section, we'll examine how we set ourselves up to fail. We actually do things that undermine our attempts to lose weight, all with the best intentions.

As we go through the book, I'll introduce various people that I've met along the way. Some of them are clients (I now coach and help others to lose weight and maintain it without dieting). Greta is trying her best, which for her is eating clean, only she can't ever stick to it. James has a high pressure job, and can't get through the afternoon without snacking. Michael finds himself devouring chocolate in the car. Maria is trying to shake off the shackles, rules and the weight that comes with her rowdy Italian family. I am grateful to everyone who allowed me to share their stories, and I'm honoured to be part of their lives. (Needless to say, all the names have been changed).

We'll see, as we go through the book, that one of the worst things you can do if you want to lose weight, is to go on a diet, or a 'healthy eating plan'. This seems completely counter-intuitive, because surely these are the very things that have been devised to solve the problem. In fact, as we'll discover, they are one of the major causes of weight gain. Shockingly, this has been known, and proven for over seventy years, but too many companies are getting rich selling diets, for anyone to admit to the fact that they don't work.

We'll examine the ways that we make it harder for ourselves to drop the weight, before exploring the many options for losing it, that work, that last, and that allow you to decide what's right for you.

Why diets make us fatter

The first time I went on a diet, I was still at school. It was all Juliette's fault - she was the cool girl in class, seventeen, with jet black hair and lashings of eyeliner. For four weeks she'd been subsisting on watermelon and vodka, when suddenly her cheekbones emerged, sharp beneath her white skin. All at once, we were all comparing bone structure.

Then Allison turned vegetarian, and at that point dieting became yet another rite of passage, a way of defining ourselves from our parents, of turning off the tap of motherly love and announcing our independence from familial food choices. None of us were fat. This was the 1980s, and obesity wasn't yet a problem.

We all lost weight. At my eighteenth birthday party, I wore a tight-fitting dress and was stunned when my relatives commented on my weight loss. I had never considered myself fat, and I had not realised, until this point, that weight loss would generate such attention, such praise and such interest. The attention made me feel special, the admiration was intoxicating.

Everyone was envious. Everyone commented. I felt powerful, sleek and sexy. But I also felt really fragile, as I didn't think I could maintain it. And I felt dangerous, not really knowing what to do with this slim new sexual body, not knowing how to cope with the envy.

I didn't have to worry because as soon as I started to eat normally, the weight came back, plus a bit more. I went to university and dieted harder. I gave up meat, then bread and pasta, then all high fat foods. Then all sugar. Until I was eating mainly vegetables and fruit. I got thin. Girls were envious. Boys were curious. I felt powerful and out of control.

Nobody could see that sometimes I got so hungry that I would just spoon peanut butter out of the jar into my mouth. Not my peanut butter either. My flat mate's.

Perhaps these compliments suck us in? I suspect that most people's first diet is a reasonably positive experience. It's novel and new and exciting and because our bodily systems haven't yet been wrecked by restriction, we usually lose weight. Often the memory of this 'first time' lingers on down the years, leading us to believe that we can recapture it, that we really can lose weight if only we try harder, because we have done so in the past. What we don't realise is that each time we diet, we make it harder and harder for ourselves. It's more likely that we'll cheat.

After a certain amount of dieting, something breaks down, and we find ourselves stuffing food into our mouths, sometimes food that we don't even like, always secretively, never at a meal, and usually washed down with a good dose of shame. A week later, we weigh more than when we started the diet. What's wrong with me, we lament. Where's my willpower? I'm fat and disgusting. I can't even control my eating. Something inside us deflates, a balloon of hope and optimism, a spark of youth extinguished. And to make sure it never lights up again, we cram in another mouthful and swallow hard.

The price of cheating is high. The price is not about the weight, although the weight is a depressing and potentially unhealthy side effect. The price of cheating is feeling terrible about yourself.

Sometimes all you lose on a diet, is hope.

We think we cheat because we are bad. Because we are failures. Because we aren't worthy. And those very thoughts make us want to give up the diets or healthy behaviours and just eat more. Every time we set out on a new healthy eating plan, we hope that it's going to be different. We hope that we will be a different person, one that sticks to the rules. And almost every time we fall short.

What if you didn't cheat because you were a bad person?

During World War Two, a group of scientists restricted the food of some perfectly healthy men for six months until they lost about 20 percent of their weight. It was called the Minnesota Starvation Experiment and sounds most unpleasant.

It was enforced dieting. As the experiment went on, these ordinary men became increasingly obsessed with food. They began to pore over recipe books. When they could eat freely, these half-starved chaps found it difficult to stop eating. They were driven by intense cravings. These symptoms didn't abate when they had regained the weight, but lasted for many many months.

This means that back in the 1940s, they had proved that dieting creates an obsession with food and an inability to stop eating once the diet is over. Science has known for over seventy years that diets don't work, and yet we are still turning to them.

Sure, you lose weight in the first instance. It's what happens afterwards that creates the problems. We're left with intense cravings and an irresistible urge to eat beyond the point of fullness. Later in the book we'll examine some of the physical mechanisms that cause this, and how to get back on track.

The diet industry is now one of the largest industries in the world. I'm including 'healthy eating' plans in this - which is the more fashionable term for diet at the moment. Worldwide, it was worth £220billion in 2017. And we are fatter than ever. Surely if diets worked, it would be a small industry: you'd go on a diet and then never need one again.

A study from Finland involving 2000 twins found that just one attempt at a diet made the twin two to three times more likely to be overweight than their non-dieting sibling.

While a UCLA review of thirty one long term studies on dieting found that dieting is a great predictor of weight GAIN (not loss). Two thirds regained more than they lost.

Diets are short term eating plans, which lead us to believe that we can return to our old behaviours and eating habits and remain thin. Dieting makes us feel as though our bodies do not know best so we hand over control to outside influences, such as the Instagram feeds or magazine articles that tell us how we should be eating. We ignore signals from our bodies – such as hunger, or tiredness in order to stick to the diet. We ignore what we want to eat and eat what we are told, sometimes things we don't really like.

We ignore when we feel hungry. And we ignore when we are not.

Soon we are so used to 'doing what we are told' that we can't tell the difference between outside influences - whether it is a diet book or an advertisement for chocolate or the window of a fast food store - and inside signals from our body.

We become programmed to respond to external stimuli rather than internal needs and lose the hunger mechanism that has kept us healthy for so long. It makes us more likely to respond to those external cues, and eat food if we so much as glimpse a photograph of it.

Maybe you're wondering if this hunger mechanism exists, or whether we are programmed to eat as much as possible as soon as presented with food. That would be logical, right? It would protect us in case of famine. I can reassure you that it does exist: there is clear evidence to show that the hunger mechanism works in all of us, as we'll see later. It also appears that it is delicate and easily over-ridden or broken. And the fastest way to over-ride or break it is with a diet.

What if the systems in your body and mind are humming like a very sophisticated machine, and you've accidentally pulled the wrong lever, a lever which leads them to betray your weight loss goals? What if there are excellent explanations for why we cheat that have nothing to do with being morally superior or inferior?

We've messed up some essential part of ourselves, and dieting is the quickest way to do this. The majority of dieters regain all the weight lost, and usually some more besides. And yet we still keep doing it. Because it seems logical, right? If you want to lose weight, then the answer is to restrict your eating.

We are left with so much emotional baggage around food and what we should be eating, that it feels very difficult to make the right decision.

The basis of this book is that there is no right decision. There is only what is right for YOU and what's right for you is likely to vary day to day and may also vary according to the time of year: many of us crave heavier food when it is colder.

By getting in touch with what you really want to eat, and stopping when your body says it is full, you will no longer feel deprived or hungry. You will be in control, rather than at the beck and call of outside forces, eating plans, Instagram feeds and books. Over time, as you work with the systems of your body, you will find that your weight returns to a healthy level without struggle.

Believe me, your body will be much better managing its weight than you have been. Sounds too good to be true?

ACTION

Make a promise to yourself that you will never diet again. Reassure your body that you will never make it eat something it doesn't want. Make a pact with yourself to start trusting your body and its needs, to start listening to it and to live in harmony with your body not at war.

Make a list of all the diets that you have been on over the year. List what you ate on each Write down how you felt on the diet Note how much weight you lost and then note how much you regained afterwards.

Notice how you feel as you think about past diets. Often the first one is a success, as we are not used to being deprived, and we seek to replicate that first time every time we diet again.

Write down how you feel about not dieting.

Summary

There are many ways that we can fool ourselves. We can eat in the car, or when no one else is looking. We can sneak a mouthful here and there. We can nibble between meals, while we feed our children or when we are clearing the dishes.

Then we can lie to ourselves and others about how much we've eaten and when. We can pretend it's healthy or that it was only a tiny bit.

It doesn't matter how we pretend to ourselves and others. The only thing we can't lie to is our bodies. They keep an accurate record of our actions. It's evident on our waists, our hips and our thighs.

Crazy Diets:
Headlines from October 2017

Victoria Beckham shows off her svelte figure in a tight polo neck... as she reveals secret to her lithe physique is drinking VINEGAR

Is Devil's Tongue the new weight loss wonder food? Obscure plant that smells of 'rotting flesh' contains ingredient that's been dubbed a 'gastric band in a glass'.

Want to know the best new way to lose weight? Just put some butter in your coffee

Simple. All you need to do is drink vinegar, put butter in your coffee and eat Devil's Tongue.
Then you'll lose weight.

CHAPTER TWO
HUNGER

In order to consider how we might go through life without cheating, we're going to have to start with hunger. Hunger may turn out to be your biggest ally, even if you might feel it's the worst thing in the world.

Not only is it worth exploring hunger, it's worth looking at the other end of the scale - satisfaction or fullness. When do we stop eating? What is enough?

Eating is the solution to hunger. Nature set us up that way. Eating wasn't intended to solve marital stress, or boredom or anger that we can't express. Non-hungry eating lies at the heart of many of our issues around food, and in order to explore that, we need to look at our nemesis - Hunger.

Hunger: friend or foe in the battle of the bulge?

For a long while I was scared of feeling hungry. Not just scared, terrified. I did everything possible to avoid hunger. In fact, there was a time when I was so scared of feeling hungry that I hadn't felt hungry for years. I never let myself get to that point.

At the very first sign that I might get a hunger pang, I'd tuck into something. At the thought that I hadn't eaten for a few hours, I'd open a packet. If I began to worry that there may be a gap between meals - I'd ensure there wasn't.

It has taken me a long time to get over that fear.

A review of the (more honest) comments of Hollywood actresses, reveals that many of them admit to feeling hungry all the time. This is the only way they can maintain their abnormally thin frames. Feeling hungry all the time can be draining and exhausting. But that is very different to feeling hungry for half an hour.

It is absolutely worth letting yourself feel hungry. If you are truly hungry when you eat, the food tastes better. There is a real sense of the body refuelling. It's the most reliable sign that your body needs to eat, rather than your head needing something to either distract it from the task at hand, prop it up through another long afternoon, or feed its addiction to sugar (of which more later).

In order to know when you're hungry, first of all you need to know what hunger feels like, and that may take a while and a little bit of courage. It means we're going to have to expose ourselves to it. This is something that you might resist, or feel reluctant to try. Remember, I'm just suggesting that you allow yourself to experience hunger - you don't have to be hungry for hours - just a few moments.

Try this on a day where you know you will be able to slake your hunger – you don't want to be ravenous in the middle of the supermarket and having to resort to ripping open confectionary in the middle of Aisle Three.... You may want to prepare a meal that you can eat when you are ready, so that you are assured of an immediate end to the hungriness, if you're particularly worried about it.

Wait until you start to get hungry and see what it feels like. If you can, sit with it for a while, and see how the feeling changes. Is it constant or does it come in waves. How does it feel physically? Do any emotions come up with the physical sensation? It might feel like some growling in the stomach. But something more than that as digestion can also feel growly. It may feel like a sense of lightness and emptiness. Prolonged hunger may accompany a feeling of tiredness, but sometimes it may energise you. Hunger may make you feel irritable and snappy. You may feel panicky at first, if it is an unfamiliar sensation. Just sit with it for a few minutes, let yourself know that you will be fed, and that it is OK to feel hungry.

Hunger can grow to be a more painful feeling in the abdomen. Some may feel it elsewhere, or as a more generalized change in their body.

I find that hunger comes and goes – it is not a constant or consistent feeling. I get hungry – some growling in the stomach, and then after about five minutes it goes away again. In about another half an hour it comes back again, but more intensely.

Sometimes I find that when I'm hungry I feel more alert (not tired which is what I expected). It's almost as if my body gives me a surge to go 'hunting' and 'kill' my prey. I feel on edge and alive. After a while, I start feeling too hungry and then shortly afterwards, irritable. So I've learned to ensure that I eat before this point.

I've also learned not to be afraid of hunger. It's not so bad. Feeling comfortable with it allows me to work with my body, and be in tune with when I need to eat. Generally, I find I can tolerate hunger in the morning, but by the end of the day, when I'm also tired, my capacity to put up with it is greatly reduced.

Other people wake up ravenous and need to eat straight away. Sometimes they feel less hungry in the evening. Neither of these is right or wrong - it's all part of learning to trust your body.

Reconnecting with your body, and your natural hunger is a key part of maintaining a healthy weight. Despite everything you've read about not trusting your body, and not having a natural stop button, you will be able to reconnect. We are all born with this facility. Small children have it. They stop eating when they have had enough and want to go and play. They haven't learned about the 'specialness' of food yet, haven't feared deprivation and restriction, haven't had their bodies disrupted by blood sugar rollercoasters, and emotional attachment to food. Their bodies have an inbuilt system that tells them when they've had enough.

We all have it - we just need to find it again.

ACTION

Be brave and seek out hunger. Wait until you really feel hungry before you eat, and if you can bear to, pause for a moment to see what hunger really feels like.

Does it feel as bad as you thought it might? Does it feel familiar? Or is it a new feeling? Do you want to get to know it a little better? Can you wait for it before you eat?

Are you hungry? Or just bored?

How hungry are you right now? Do you know? How hungry were you when you ate breakfast this morning? Or when you ate lunch? How much of your food is consumed when you are actually hungry?

Research shows that in overweight people, non-hungry eating can account for as much as a hundred percent of their eating. That means, that they never wait until they are hungry, they never know what hunger feels like.

Do you blame them?

Hunger is not supposed to be a pleasant sensation. Nature designed us so that we are motivated to quell the feelings of hunger. It is a basic survival instinct. However, feeling hunger for a few minutes is not so bad. In fact, it can be quite a revelation.

Boredom is another uncomfortable feeling, and what better way to avoid it, than with a constant stream of snacks. Shortly after my stint in the chocolate factory, I found myself working in the marketing department. You might hope that temptation was further away, but the office had a staff shop and every day I would buy a packet of sugary treats to get me through the day. Any time that I felt at a loose end, frustrated or bored, I'd open the drawer of my desk, usually pretending that I was looking for a stapler or paperclip, and sneak a sweet into my mouth.

Eating when we're bored is a great way to pass the time. It's also a way of coping when we're struggling with a task. Yesterday, I was sitting at my desk, wrestling with a sentence and before I knew what I was doing, I found myself on my feet, wandering towards the kitchen. It makes me smile that even today, part of me wants to go and rifle through the refrigerator rather than sit and face what is uncomfortable. In the end I went for a walk, and eventually the rhythm of my feet helped the words flow.

If you're eating when you're bored, it can be difficult to decide what you are hungry for and what you feel like eating, because you are not actually hungry.

Sometimes it can be difficult to know whether you are hungry or thirsty, particularly if you have spent many years adhering to detoxes or diets or rule books. Notice where in your body you feel the discomfort – is your mouth dry or your body temperature changing? Lack of water can affect our temperature, energy levels and mood.

Whilst its important to stay hydrated, we can do this with tea and other hot drinks. We don't have to drink eight glasses of water a day. This oft-quoted figure was taken from a study that included, in the eight glass estimate, water in food - such as soup, in fruits and so on. Recent research is showing that many drinks, including tea, can be just as hydrating as water. Even if these drinks have a diuretic effect (ie they cause your body to lose water) if you are dehydrated, these drinks still replenish your fluid levels.

Sugary drinks, such as fruit juice, smoothies, soft drinks and alcohol are another things altogether - they are loaded with sugar that will set off a whole host of other issues as we'll see later.

Distinguishing between hunger and emotions can be a tricky one. I reckon it took me about fifteen years to tell the difference. I spent the first ten believing that I couldn't possibly be eating for emotional reasons. I didn't feel emotional, I just wanted to eat...

The majority of us eat at one time or another to satisfy emotional needs, rather than the physical need for food. Healthy eating plans and diets don't factor in arguments with loved ones, stressful days at work or boredom.

People can eat from many emotions including:

- Anger
- Stress
- Loneliness
- Boredom
- Celebration
- Grief

Try to work out whether it is emotions that are driving you to eat. The easiest way to often to think of something plain, like toast or an apple and see if you want that. If you only really want 'forbidden' foods – odds are that you aren't hungry.

The process of eating is a complex chemical and physiological process in our bodies and can provide comfort, warmth and relaxation when we need it. Some emotional eating is natural. It becomes a problem when the hunger instinct is absent from a large proportion of eating.

ACTION
Wait until you feel hungry and then notice how it feels. Sit with it for 30 minutes and write down the physical and emotional changes that come over you. How does it feel?

Are you hungry, or is it just lunch-o-clock?

Most people assume that because it's lunch time, that they should have something to eat. They crack open a sandwich and start eating, with no regard to hunger or whether they are ready to eat.

Maybe you think I'm crazy to even mention it - of course they should eat! It's lunch time!

In reality, meal times have varied greatly over history. Our rules about when we eat are relatively new. Breakfast is a modern invention, arriving sometime in the 17th century. Before then, people didn't eat in the morning. From Roman times to Middle Ages, everyone ate in the middle of the day and often it was the only meal. This is still the case for Buddhist monks, who eat a single meal at noon. The evening meal, by comparison, has long been a more sociable one, and this has become later and later with the advent of electric light. In Spain, dinner isn't served until 10pm which is agonisingly overdue for many of us.

If meal times are arbitrary and culturally determined, perhaps you can set your own?

You may also find that your body naturally gets hungry at certain times of day. I don't feel hungry first thing in the morning, and find eating breakfast makes me feel sluggish and sleepy. I get hungry at around 9.30 or 10am. There is no reason that I can't breakfast at that time. When I've worked in offices, I've packed something and taken it in. Other days I don't feel hungry until late morning, so I skip breakfast and have an early lunch.

It might suit you to have a late lunch at 2pm - when you're hungry and when it will see you through until dinner. It's hard to know unless you've been brave enough to break some of the rules and find out.

There is also no evidence that skipping a meal does you any harm whatsoever. In fact, sometimes, giving your digestive system a break, allows your body to work on healing itself, and getting itself back into balance.

It can be quite scary to miss a meal. You may find yourself checking in every few minutes to see whether you are hungry, or worrying that you will run out of energy. It can be a nice surprise to find that your body will work without a constant drip feed of food, that you can survive a few hours on your own. You may find that discovery empowering.

Part of trusting yourself, and learning when to eat when hungry, is giving yourself permission to explore these ideas. Some of them may seem confronting, especially if they go against cultural and social norms. Not eating lunch until 3pm, when everyone around you is eating it at 1pm can be challenging. You may find, however, that this works for you and allows you to remain energised until dinner. You won't find out until you try.

ACTION

Wait until you are hungry before eating, even if this means delaying a meal.

Experiment with eating at different times of day, or moving meals a little earlier or later and see how you feel.

Find what times would suit you to eat (work and family permitting). Are there times that you naturally feel hungry or want to eat?

Have we forgotten what 'full' feels like?

Full is.... Feeling the vomit rising in the back of my throat when I just can't get another thing down..... Having to loosen the button on my jeans and lie down.... Never wanting to eat again...Full is that feeling after Christmas lunch.

Or is it?

Perhaps it's that feeling of the hunger fading and a nice relaxed sensation stealing over me? Maybe 'Full' is the sensation of rumbling subsiding, my body being sated, and my stomach being comfortable.

Our stomachs are not like the petrol tanks in our cars. There isn't a little dial that hits the top and we stop. Our stomachs are, in reality, like an elastic bag, able to shrink or balloon. This means the notion of full is hard to define.

We've lost touch with what satisfied feels like. Too many diets, too many big meals, too many meals eaten in front of the television or in the car. We have forgotten when to stop eating.

When are we satisfied? When is too much, not enough?

For a long while, I thought, genuinely, that full meant a feeling of discomfort. I believed that full meant, as in a car, that you couldn't physically fit anything else in. As a definition – that is what full is in other circumstances. But full is an uncomfortable thing. I was often uncomfortable at the end of a meal, or, if I wasn't, I'd often continue eating chocolate or other food until I felt that way. And of course, with that feeling comes the guilt. Not to mention the kilos....

Back in 1990, scientists gave dieters a pudding - one group is told it is high calorie, another group that it is low calorie. (This strikes me as pretty dishonest, given that it's the same pudding every time.)

The dieters eat far more when they believe it to be high calorie than when they are told it is low calorie. Perception that the diet is broken seems to be more important than the actual calories consumed. People who aren't chronic dieters don't do this: they eat less if they think that it's more fattening.

This is one of many pieces of research that shows that the very people who are trying the hardest to lose weight eat more when they know it's going to damage their diet the most. The puddings don't taste any different. They don't feel any more or less full. It's all in the mind. It's about blowing the diet. If you've messed up the diet, then you go gangbusters and eat like it's an Olympic sport. I know. I've done it.

But if there's no diet - you can't blow it. Which is why losing touch with our bodies is so catastrophic. We're no longer in tune with what we do and don't want, only with what we can't have, or don't allow ourselves to have. If we allow ourselves food, perhaps we might know when to stop, when we feel satisfied.

Sometimes it's not an impending diet that throws us. Sometimes we can eat a whole meal and not feel satisfied. Maybe you really wanted a large plate of creamy pasta with mushrooms, but told yourself that you 'should' have a salad with chicken

So, you eat the salad with chicken, and gradually fill up, but you don't feel satisfied. Some part of you still wants the creamy pasta, even after a salad

Of the people I have met over the years, Greta is typical of so many of us who take our health seriously and try to do the right things. Greta has been focused on "eating clean" for the past few years. She's really careful about what she can and can't eat during the week. Then, on the weekends, she "does ok for breakfast and lunch" then "it all goes to hell at "dinner" with bread, a large meal, dessert, and alcohol, if she goes out with friends. If she has a weekend in, which she sometimes does, just to avoid going out and eating too much, she finds herself eating 'forbidden' foods all weekend. She'll open a bag of cookies to find she's scoffed the lot.

Then she's filled with guilt. By Monday, she feels like a failure, feels ugly, beats herself up, and renews her commitment to eat even "cleaner" and restrict even more. The cycle repeats almost every week to the point where she feels like once she starts eating treats, it's like she can't stop. She feels frustrated and stuck, and as though her body is her enemy.

When we discussed what she ate for lunch, she responded that she had a quinoa and kale salad. (Right on trend, I thought. Gwyneth would be proud of you). We started talking about whether she felt satisfied after this, and she eventually admitted that she didn't. She might feel full, but not that satisfied. In fact, when she thought back, she had enjoyed the salad the first couple of times she bought it, but now she ate it because she thought she 'should' rather than because she chose to, and she'd stopped enjoying it.

Greta committed to make an effort to really think about what she wanted to eat during the week, and for a while, quinoa and kale really wasn't it. She gave herself permission to eat other choices. At first it was other salads, she wasn't brave enough to try a wrap or a sandwich as she was worried about the carbohydrates. She agreed to have one, on a day when she really craved it, and she found that over time, her weekend overeating subsided, because she allowed herself more satisfying food during the week. She also found, that after a few weeks, she craved a kale and quinoa salad and enjoyed it.

The only way for her to get off the cycle was to stop believing that 'one last time' on a strict plan would fix everything. She had to break the cycle, and the only way to break it was by giving herself permission to eat. Greta had to take the terrifying step of trusting herself.

It's very easy to get into a rut where we limit our food choices. It can feel safe that way, as though we are in control. This is often linked to not trusting ourselves or our bodies. There may be some justification for this in the case of highly processed foods - we will see later in the book how they can trigger over-eating whether we like it or not. But if we are limiting ourselves to a very small range of foods, and are anxious about eating an entire food group (such as carbohydrates) then it's worth expanding our options.

You may feel apprehensive about branching out and eating a wider range of foods. Once again, it's something to do in your own time, and when your body is asking for something. You may find that you are ready to test some of the 'rules' that have bound you, a time that you feel able to question your restrictions, and ask yourself what you'd really like to eat.

Satisfaction is an important part of weight management. We don't always give ourselves permission to be satisfied, to be content. It's all part of the rushing and self-denial that is on trend. Not many of us admit to sitting down and enjoying our food, allowing ourselves to feel delighted, to feel as though we are nurtured.

If you feel nurtured and satisfied by your meal, it's unlikely you will want to cheat. Satisfied has a different ring about it to full. It has a lot of different connotations. It's about having your senses pleased. It's about various appetites – not just hunger – it's about being satisfied with the appearance of the food, with the place that you're eating. If you're in a restaurant it's about the service and the company. You can have a great meal and not feel satisfied. Maybe it wasn't what you wanted to eat? Or maybe it was but the conversation was upsetting. Maybe the food was lovely, but it was cold. Or perhaps it used to be your favourite thing and it has disappointed you. Satisfaction depends on so many things.

Maria says: "For me, satisfaction might mean just a taste of something: a mouthful of a salty strong cheese, or a snapped fragment of dark rich chocolate. Other times I might need a large, warming, comforting bowl of nourishing pasta to heat me from the core. Or a crisp cool slice of melon on a hot day. It's hard to cheat if you feel satisfied. Satisfaction has a contentedness to it, a sated feeling. A sense that I've had exactly what I need."

'Full' doesn't feel like that. It's stuffed, without thought or care. It's about quantity not quality and usually means that it's uncomfortable physically - bloating, draining, lethargic.

Tuning in to what will make us satisfied means listening to our bodies and minds. It relies on listening to the various signals from your stomach, your palate. This takes time, in a world where we are always rushing to drop the kids, grab a sandwich, get to the bus. So we forego the time to work out what we'd really like, what would satisfy us, and cram something easy down instead.

Learning when to stop eating is a key part of getting back in tune with your natural appetite. Each time you eat more than your body needs, it's going to shunt the extra off to fat.

One of the loveliest things I heard from a client was: 'Today, full is what I feel when joy fills me up. A smile from a friend, a small kindness. These make me feeling more full than food ever did or could.'

ACTION

Try keeping a hunger diary where you record how hungry or satisfied you are throughout the day. Notice when you feel satisfied. Is that different to feeling full?

Summary

Allowing yourself to overcome any fear or trepidation about hunger, and gradually to feel comfortable with it, is one of the most important steps to stop cheating around food.

Feeling hungry at least once is day is normal. It means that we are ready for a meal. If we aren't hungry, then perhaps we need to wait a little longer before we eat.

Distinguishing between hunger and thirst and hunger and emotions might be difficult at first. This is something that will become easier the more you allow yourself to feel hunger. Its energising growl is quite unmistakeable.

You may want to experiment with meal times, to find the best times for you to eat. Portion size, either reducing or increasing it, might tide you over better between meals or ensure that you are hungry enough for the next one.

Once you have eaten, working out when you've had enough is something else that only your body can tell you. No packet, or diet, or recipe can predict what will be sufficient for you. Only you know that, and it's likely to vary day by day.

The most important skill we can develop for health weight management, is to get in tune with our hunger and satisfaction.

CHAPTER THREE
PHYSIOLOGICAL REASONS

It's becoming clear that one of the most important things that we need to do is get back in tune with our bodies and their natural rhythms of hunger and satisfaction. However, there are a number of physiological events and processes that make this harder for us.

We can trigger certain hormonal systems that increase hunger and appetite, which won't work in our favour. This leaves us wanting to eat lots of sugary foods, reliant on willpower to stop us, which isn't a desirable situation.

However, different behaviours can generate a sense of fullness that lasts longer, and diminishes cravings. We'll look at the importance of fat, protein and carbohydrates and examine in more detail sugar and sugar substitutes. Gluten and food intolerances are also covered, together with the latest research in these area.

Factors such as stress and sleep play a role, as do our gut bacteria. All of these react and interplay to affect our hunger levels and our weight.

An understanding of how we can make life easier for ourselves, allows us to make more informed choices about how we eat and when.

Sugar and Insulin: a rollercoaster

"I find sugar craving worse than hunger. Hunger is an energising growl in the stomach, an empty feeling that can be sated. Sugar cravings itch in your veins, they make me restless, twitchy, irritable and sour. I long for sweetness to sweeten my mood, to calm the jumpiness that gets me out of my chair, hunting for something to salve the prickling under my skin, to soothe the part of me that craves relief."

Mary, 43

Sugar. Delicious sprinkled on strawberries and cream or "pure, white and deadly"? As addictive as cocaine? Or the perfect ingredient for icing on a birthday cake?

Sugar has been blamed for everything from tooth decay to obesity. It's currently the chief suspect for many diseases from Alzheimers to Diabetes. Yet it's in so many of the things that we eat, particularly those things that we love.

I'm quite partial to it. I love the way that the tartness of lemon is lifted by a sugary cloud of meringue. I adore the caramelized richness that a pinch of sugar will give to slowly cooking onions. I love the childhood memories that flood back at the first taste of liquorice (especially dipped in sherbet).

It's only natural. We are programmed to like sugar. Our very first taste, of breast milk, is actually slightly sweet. This, combined with the fat in the milk is a seductive introduction to the pleasures of food. If you've ever seen a baby after it's been fed, it looks almost drunk on the heady combination. From the word go, we are primed to enjoy it.

But we're a very clever species and we've worked out how to isolate the sweet taste without any of the accompanying fibre and vitamins that nature so carefully includes: fibre and vitamins that our bodies need. It's what sugar does to our body when it's stripped of all these vitamins and fibre that undermines us. It undermines us in several ways, driving us to eat more because:

- It stimulates the hormone insulin which leads to fat storage
- It increases appetite
- It's addictive

When we eat sugar, our body produces insulin, a hormone which allows us to deal with it. The problem with this, is that one of insulin's main functions is to store fat. So the more insulin we produce, the more likely we are to store fat. Therefore the more sugar we eat, the more of the fat-storing hormone (insulin) we generate. Not a great start.

All carbohydrates, not just sugar, lead us to produce insulin. Some carbs, like oats, or sweet potatoes, take more work to get them into the blood stream, so the insulin drips out slowly to match the release from the gut. But a stonking great hit of processed sugary food leads to a massive injection of insulin.

The body then worries that it's made too much insulin and over compensates by releasing already digested sugar in the form of glucose. This is because too much insulin - which lowers blood sugar, can lead to a coma. In fact too much sugar in the blood can also lead to a coma, which is why insulin is such a critical hormone and why diabetes is so dangerous.

Our current way of eating, with a lot of highly processed carbohydrates, means that we are constantly pumped with insulin. It's very easy to get onto the sugar rollercoaster. You get a sugar rush, then you hit an insulin low, so you need more sugar to make you feel better. Sugar cravings are then mistaken for hunger. They will get you hunting for food way faster than hunger, and they can be far more uncomfortable.

But they do feel different.

Hunger starts in the stomach, with an emptiness, a growling. Sugar starts more in the head, or the limbs, a tickling or craving. A need for something. If you're on a sugar and insulin rollercoaster, it's going to be hard not to cheat. At least, it's going to be hard until you get your blood sugar under control.

James has a high pressure job in a law firm, and usually skips breakfast, firing up his system with a large coffee. By mid morning, he is hungry and grabs a pastry. The mixture of sugar and white flour flood his body and he feels instantly better. But an hour later, he feels flat again, driven to seek out something to pep him up.

When he came to see me, he was 'medicating himself' almost every hour with either caffeine or sugar to keep himself going. Lunch was a packet of crisps or a sandwich and then in the afternoon, he'd snack on chocolate to prevent the terrible slumps of exhaustion that would strike him down if he didn't.

We discussed ways that he might be able to level out his blood sugar. He wasn't hungry first thing, so we agreed that skipping breakfast wasn't a problem, but he would need something to stabilise his blood sugar mid morning. In the end, we settled on a can of tuna, protein being one of the best things to maintain even blood sugar levels.

It was easy for James to stack his office drawer with cans of tuna and he liked the links with body building diets, which seem to be built around cans of tuna, rice and protein shakes. He kept meaning to get more into serious weight-lifting, if only his job wasn't so busy. Within a week, he felt different. The tuna stopped the sugar train in its tracks. He wasn't so hungry at lunch time, when again, he made sure he had a sandwich, with plenty of protein. James still sometimes eats chocolate in the afternoon, but because this time, he wants it, not because he can't function without it.

He lost ten kilograms, he says 'without trying'. In reality, he did try. He tried something new - eating some tuna mid-morning. This worked with his body and with his blood sugar and helped him function better to the point where he felt he was still making sharp decisions at the end of the afternoon when he would have previously felt groggy and tired.

Sugar is a very easy substance to use as a pick-me-up when you're feeling tired or down because it gives you an energy boost. When you start down this track, it's common to want increasing quantities. I find that if I have a little sugar one week, the next week I want more, until I realise that my intake is growing along with my waistline. The more sugar you have, the more you want. Your palate adapts and seeks out sweeter tasting things. Foods that might have been sweet enough on their own, like fruit, start to feel as though they need something extra. Then before you know it, you're sprinkling sugar on everything. Worse still, your body adapts to regular sugar intake, and starts to crave the stuff.

Sugar is also very easy to consume in relatively large quantities. It doesn't make you feel full or satisfied and an hour or so later, you're ready for some more. Worse, if you want to increase your appetite, sugar is a sure fire way.

Sugar makes you more hungry so that you eat more. This is partly due to the insulin high and low that sugar induces. This starts your body on a hunger cycle even if it doesn't require food – the insulin peaks and troughs make you believe you're ravenous even when you have plenty of food to burn.

If you eat sugary things: soft drinks, sweets, biscuits – not only will these things not fill you up, they are likely to make you eat more of other foods and feel famished.

I'm not a fan of cutting out food groups - all the research shows this backfires. Eliminating it completely leaves us with the psychological difficulties that an restriction brings - as you'll see later.

So let's approach this with caution. Just as fat was completely vilified in the 1980s and 1990s, now it's sugar's turn. While it's clear that eating a large amount of sugar is damaging to your health, a spoonful of brown sugar on your porridge isn't going to hurt you.

Finding a moderate way is far harder than the all-or-nothing approach. It means we each need to work out what's right for us. We'll see other ways that we can do this in the following chapters.

More than anything, it's going to be hard to control your weight, or resist temptation while your blood sugar is all over the place. So the more you can do to get that nice and stable, the better.

ACTION

Try to be aware of how sugar makes you feel.

Does it make you hungrier? Do you want more when you eat more? Notice how you feel when you eat something sweet – both immediately afterwards, and thirty minutes later.

Were sweet things used as a reward in your family?

How much sugar would you choose to eat in a day?

Sugar substitutes: worse than the real thing

Artificial sweeteners might look like a godsend - a way to have the sweet taste without the calories, whether it's aspartame or saccharin. But new research shows it's not as simple as this. Several studies show consuming low-calorie artificial sweeteners make you more likely to pile on weight than reduce it.

Our bodies are expecting sugar when we taste something sweet, so the insulin roller coaster sets off, whether we like it or not and whether we eat sugar or not. The sweetness on our tongue is all that's required. Our brains are expecting the dopamine hit it normally gets from sugar (more of that in the next section), except that it doesn't arrive. Which means that we can crave sweet things or carbohydrates even more, after eating artificial sweeteners. This stands true even of the more 'natural' low calorie sweeteners such as Stevia.

So rather than helping us consume less sugar overall, because they interfere with our satisfaction signals, artificial sweeteners cause us to crave even more sweet food. A study in the United States showed that while people who drank one to two cans of full-sugar fizzy drinks a day increased their risk of becoming overweight or obese by nearly 33 per cent over seven to eight years, those who replaced them with diet alternatives had a 65 per cent risk. It strikes me as extraordinary that you're twice as likely to get fat on diet drinks.

'Natural' sweeteners such as honey, agave syrup and plant extracts such as stevia are now being touted as better for you than sugar.

The truth is somewhat less palatable. Both refined and unrefined sugars have much the same effect on the body. While refined table sugar (sucrose) is dealt with by the pancreas (which produces insulin), unrefined fruit sugars are processed by the liver. Despite this biochemical difference, our bodies react to unrefined, natural sweeteners in much same way as a spoonful of the white stuff – with a blood sugar spike. This encourages the liver to produce glucose, and high blood glucose levels ultimately cause the body to store fat and gain weight.

Products containing fructose contribute to obesity, heart problems and liver disease just like products containing granulated sugar. It may even drain minerals from your body. Alternative sugars are also implicated in weight gain and tooth decay; they also perpetuate our taste for sweet things – because many are actually sweeter than sugar.

Some options, like honey are higher in calories than table sugar. A tablespoon of commercial natural honey contains 64 calories whereas a tablespoon of sugar contains around 48 calories.

Agave is a favourite sweetener of clean-eating bloggers. It is made from a fluid extracted from blue agave, a native Mexican plant that is also used to make tequila. This fact was almost enough to make me want to try it, but then I discovered that the juice is filtered, heated and concentrated, meaning it is highly processed, just like sugar, and marketed as a "nectar". It's up to 90 per cent fructose, and high in calories too, at 60 per tablespoon.

Brown rice syrup is fructose free. This is because, it is 100 per cent glucose, so consumption leads to a massive blood sugar spike. Additionally, it's processed. Brown rice syrup is made from fermented cooked brown rice boiled into syrup that completely removes any nutrients, leaving behind only glucose. Not only is this empty calories (75 per tbsp), but it's also the highest scoring sweetener on the GI index (98).

A brief aside on the Glycemic Index (GI). This is a measure of how fast sugar hits our blood stream. It's a useful way to see how quickly we'll get a sugar hit, and can help us manage our blood sugar by eating 'low GI'. Under 50 is low GI.

Stevia is 'sweet' on the palate, so the body assumes it is receiving sugar and primes itself to do so. Glucose is cleared from the bloodstream and blood sugars drop, but no real sugar/glucose is provided to the body to compensate. Insulin rises rapidly. In fact, recent research shows that Stevia can raise insulin levels to such a degree that it may assist diabetics whose insulin pathways no longer function. Given that we are trying to minimise insulin spikes, in order to keep our blood sugar under control, these findings make me wary of Stevia.

Whether it is labelled as 'healthy' or 'natural' or low calorie, sweet is sweet as far as our bodies are concerned. They all generate an insulin rush, They can all lead to weight gain (especially, it seems, the ones with no calories... go figure.)

It's worth considering them all as much the same, whether honey, maple syrup, molasses, aspartame or sugar. If you want something sweet, then one might not be that much better than another. So have pancakes with maple syrup, or a cake made with sugar. Or have a real bounty bar rather than the 'healthy bounty bars' so beautifully crushed by Catherine Saxelby in the section on 'but it was healthy'.

If you really want something sweet, then have it. Have it and enjoy it.

ACTION

As Michael Pollan so eloquently puts it in his book 'In Defence of Food': 'watch out for those health claims'.

Be aware that any sweet taste is going to trigger an insulin response. Would you rather have sugar? Or can you do without it?

Notice how you feel after sugar. Do you feel better? Does your mood change? Do you find that you crave it more over the following days or does having a little of it satisfy you?

Protein: the friend you never knew you had

Mary had been a vegetarian for a decade and had put on a lot of weight. She didn't really like pulses and so, although she ate a lot of vegetables, her meals tended not to have a great deal of protein. By the time she came to see me, she was craving carbs, and would find herself eating vast quantities of bread or rice with butter and cheese, unable to sate her hunger.

Having been vegetarian for a few years myself, I sympathised. I had found myself in a similar situation, and it took a nutritionist to persuade me that I might be craving protein. Don't get me wrong - I'm highly supportive of vegetarian and vegan diets - most of us eat too much meat which has shown to be detrimental to our health.

Mary agreed to eat more protein. She included eggs in her meals and said that she could eat fish occasionally. Within a month, she had lost weight.

Protein can do amazing things for your body. It provides all those vital nutrients that help rebuild your muscles, your skin, and your hair. It is vital for good health, strong bones and muscles and for your cells to regenerate.

But more importantly, protein can do wonderful things for your appetite. Just as sugar can make you hungrier, protein will reduce your appetite. This is largely due to its stabilising effect on blood sugar. Protein, especially eaten at every meal, will keep your blood sugar levels steady and consistent and when these stop fluctuating, you'll stop having hunger pangs so often. Your mood will be more reasonable. Your emotions will calm down as your whole system is more regulated.

Protein doesn't necessarily mean meat. Personally, I'm not a big meat eater. It might mean eggs, ricotta (delicious for breakfast or even a sweet treat with fruit), nuts, and yoghurt. Of course it may be fish, ham, chicken or beef. Even a small amount with every meal will make a large difference to the way you feel and your hunger levels.

This is one of the issues with juice fasts and detoxes that only include fruit and vegetables - they mess up your blood sugar. It's impossible to feel sane on them as there is no protein to keep you full. You're setting yourself up to cheat.

Eating protein regularly also helps protect your muscle mass. Without protein, your body cannibalises its own muscles stores. The last thing you want to do is lose muscle, as muscle burns calories even when we aren't doing anything with them. You'll look like you're losing weight, as the scales will be going down, but if you're burning muscle rather than fat, your metabolism is going to drop, and of course then, you will put on weight even if you reduce your calorie intake. Not the best scenario...

Research has shown that eating more protein can itself give us a metabolic boost. A high protein, moderate carb diet burns around 4 percent more calories more than a high carb moderate protein one - not a huge amount but it all helps. The subjects of the higher protein diet reported lower hunger and a significant increase in fullness. All things that we'd like.

Bodybuilders know all of this - they build their diets around regular protein. I'm not suggesting that we become body builders, but they are competing to be as lean as possible - and they know a trick or two.

ACTION
See if you can incorporate more protein into your diet, while still eating foods you enjoy.

Crazy Diets: Alas Smith and Jones

Griff: It's called the Beverley Hills H Bomb diet. Every day I have to eat a specific amount of things.

Mel: What kind of things? Tiny things?

Griff: Oh God yeah, tiny. Like really tiny. Tiny things. This is my fifth day.

Mel: Right. What have you got to eat today then?

Griff: I dunno.

Mel: You dunno?

Griff: I ate the book I was so hungry

Cutting out fat: is that a good thing or not?

Low fat, high fibre diets were all the rage in the 70s. There was the famous F Plan which seemed to consist mainly of baked potatoes and baked beans. (One of my mother's friends called it the fart plan). It was an inexpensive way to eat and this may have fitted with the much tighter household budgets of that decade. Rosemary Conley reinvigorated this approach in the UK in the 1990s with her Hip and Thigh Diet.

I tried to stick to low fat eating for a while. I ate large quantities of cottage cheese, an ingredient that I found unpalatable even back then. I would mix all kinds of things into it to make it edible, settling eventually on tomato ketchup, which rendered it a soft peach pink. I fondly imagined that it might be like the creamy and tart Marie Rose sauce in which prawn cocktails are drenched, but anyone looking at my plate, at the lumpy pink mess wouldn't be fooled. And, to be frank, neither was I. The manufacturers must have caught on, as they started selling cottage cheese with pineapple. Everyone knows that when you add acidic fruit to dairy you get a curdled mess. But as that's pretty much what cottage cheese is to start with, so I guess it didn't matter.

I haven't touched it since.

Low fat diets were one of the first crazes to sweep our modern dieting world. Since then, there have been many variations on this theme by many authors. All of them maintain that if you cut out fat you will lose weight. There is some truth in the theory that if we eat less fat, we'll lose weight. Large amounts of fat once eaten, do have a tendency to deposit themselves on the body. Not what we're looking for.

Fat is high in calories and easy to over consume. Logically, reducing your intake, is likely to reduce your weight. But that isn't necessarily true. If you merely replace fat with sugary foods, then you will NOT lose weight. You will land back on the insulin rollercoaster, an unenviable ride of mood swings and cravings that lead only to the biscuit cupboard.

This is what many food manufacturers have done. Because removing the fat often removes the taste, or at least much of the pleasure, something needs to be done to make the food palatable. The easiest fix is to slap a load of sugar in. It's a surprising fact that many low fat foods have as many calories as their higher fat equivalents, sometimes more. And while I don't advocate calorie counting, neither do I advocate swapping fat calories for sugar ones. That's just bonkers.

Low fat eating can end up being high glycemic – which means that blood sugar starts peaking and dipping, which makes it hard to feel satisfied for long. Baked potatoes for example, are high glycemic – which means that the energy from them enters the blood stream very quickly, giving you a nice 'rush' and satisfied feeling, which is followed 30-60 minutes later by a feeling that maybe you didn't eat enough after all. This energy crash can then inspire immediate and urgent chocolate cravings.

I met Laura at the gym - she loves working out and she covets the ultra-ripped, lean look that's in a lot of the fitness magazines. Her diet was already strict - she had cut out sugar, she ate no junk. But despite this, and despite her arduous workouts, she still couldn't attain the low levels of body fat needed to imitate the photographs she admired.

So she cut out all fat. She wasn't eating much in the first place, but out went salmon and avocado. Salads were eaten without dressing, nothing was fried. With the fat went a lot of the flavour and enjoyment. It took about two weeks of this before the cracks started to show. Her sugar cravings shot through the roof, and she started drizzling honey on her chicken, in an attempt to get taste or moisture. A few days later, she fell off the bandwagon and into a vat of ice cream.

Laura said that she knew the photos in magazines were photoshopped, and she understood that most of these fitness models take some form of drug or steroid to become that lean but it didn't stop her wanting to look like that, or feeling as though they represented some standard that she should live up to. Cutting out fat was the final straw. Her body, her palate, her whole being rebelled.

When I think of low fat eating I think of two things: sustainability and health. For sustainability, I wonder if I could go the rest of my life without cheese? The answer is clear. I think not. I love minestrone soup - which is a healthy bowl of vegetables, but I only love it with Parmesan thickly sprinkled on it. And as for the cheese boards when I go to my friend Heather's house? I'm certainly not abstaining from those.

Bread is supposed to have butter on it (or avocado, or peanut butter). Otherwise you'll end up like poor William Banting, who we'll meet next, who resorted to 'a tablespoon of spirit' to make his dry toast edible.

Then there is health. Ingredients like olive oil and avocados are great for your body. We're encouraged to eat 'oily' fish. On the other hand, eating lots of cream, butter and fried food is not going to be good for your health or your waistline. Whereas olive oil, nuts, avocado, oily fish have fats that are essential for cell function. So including them in your daily diet makes a lot of sense.

As for the higher fat things – work out which ones you really enjoy. Think about when you'd like to eat them most of all and then make sure that you savour a wonderful piece of Roquefort (drizzled with honey as they do in Rome), or a scoop of ice cream – when you really want them, and when they call to you like a nightingale from the stars.

Giving up fat is a sure path to cheating. Our bodies need it.

Low carb: why it isn't the miracle you hope

Low carb diets are a relatively new idea that have garnered huge momentum. As with most diets, there are some who have achieved astounding weight loss through adhering to their stark and demanding regimes.

Most include unlimited amounts of steak, chicken and fish accompanied by green vegetables and nothing else. Even fruit is off limits. Breakfast is likely to be eggs, but no oats or toast. The mystery as to why people lose weight on these diets is relatively easy to solve. They are eating far fewer calories. It's almost impossible to overeat such a limited array of food.

One of the first consequences of such a diet is a slowing of the digestive process. The body is not getting the fibre it needs (which is usually obtained from whole grains, fruit skins and so on). And let's face it, constipation is not one of life's sexier aspects.

Then there is the mind-numbing slog of meal after meal of steak or chicken and green salad. It gets pretty boring pretty quickly. Add to this, 'that specific hunger that comes with avoiding carbs', to quote Gwyneth Paltrow, and you have a recipe for misery, boredom, constipation, hunger... and eventually you will crack, like a prisoner who can take no more.

Our bodies were designed to be omnivorous (just like our closest relatives, the apes). Even our hunter gatherer ancestors ate carbohydrates. Paleo man would find a bee's nest and gorge on the honey. When fruit was in season they would eat their fill. Let's face it: they were pretty desperate. They ate loads of things we wouldn't even contemplate today. (The Hunter Gatherer and Paleo Diet seem conveniently to forget this. Instead you'll find recipes for blueberry expresso brownies. I somehow think that our ancestors weren't chowing down on those round the campfire.)

The more extreme low-carb diets recommend something called Ketosis. This is where there is no fuel for the body to burn so it breaks down its own fat stores. In order to generate this state, even protein has to be cut down. 70 percent of calories must come from fat, with the remainder from protein. Effectively you have to munch through large wads of butter without anything to put it on. The entire insulin mechanism is turned off and only fat is burned. Whilst this might sound desirable, the side effects of Ketosis are low energy, headaches, bad breath and nausea. Not exactly pleasant. Research has shown there is no metabolic boost. If you add a small amount of carbs to the same diet your metabolism would run four percent higher. Added to which, let's face it, it would be hell. Of course you'd cheat!

However, there are benefits to increasing protein intake and reducing carbohydrates. Doctors are seeing reduced cholesterol and blood pressure. Body builders, who live and die by how lean they can get for a competition, understand that carbs are necessary, but reducing them can reduce your fat levels but even they do so in moderation (they do other crazy things, don't you worry.)

Do you really want to live your life never having another birthday cake? Do you really want to refuse the bread basket or chocolate for the rest of your life? Thought not. Me neither.

So let's take the good out of the research: there is benefit in having a lower consumption of carbohydrate. Lowering how many carbs we eat helps to keep our blood sugar stable, and diminishes cravings. Our diet has become very carb heavy with all the developments in food processing and the availability of fast food, confectionery and other snacks. We could all do with watching how much we eat, particularly of carbohydrate and ensuring that a moderate amount only is consumed. But I don't think we need to give it up forever!

It's very tempting take one piece of research and hail it as the answer and then take it to extreme. If I have found nothing else during my years of research into this topic, it is that there isn't one answer. We are such complicated beings, made up of a complex physiology, brains that think, memories, cultures and hormones that no single thing is the solution.

It's much easier to sell a diet book with a single, simple idea. Much easier than admitting that the reality is complicated.

So what then do we eat and how much and when? This isn't a book that prescribes specifics, because we are each individual, and we all have different preferences and needs. One idea that we can throw out is that carbs shouldn't be eaten after a certain time. Some people refuse to eat carbs after 4pm, certain that it has helped them lose weight. The truth is, it probably has, and if this way of eating suits you, then do it. Others, me included, really like carbs in the evening. They help me relax, and I often want something comforting and substantial at the end of the day.

This isn't a ticket for weight gain. Our bodies respond to the total number of calories and total number of nutrients. For the time of day to have any impact on our body composition, everything else has to be so perfect, that it's only really worth looking at timing of food if you are a competitive body builder. Otherwise, eat carbs when you want them.

It is worth keeping an eye on the glycemic index of what you're eating as this can help with both cravings and weight control. Carbs can spike blood sugar, and the ones that do so less, such as, for example, sweet potato, basmati rice and barley, allow us to avoid insulin peaks and troughs, and therefore feel fuller longer and less at the mercy of sugar cravings. Needless to say, the more processed carbs, such as white bread, crackers and cakes hit our bloodstream much faster.

There are other benefits to wholegrains, other than the fact that their fibre keeps us fuller longer and levels out our energy. They are good for our gut and the bacteria that live there, as we'll see in the section on 'but my micro biome told me to'.

Otherwise, try playing with portion size. Just cutting down how much we are eating of a certain thing can make a far bigger difference than we realise. Having an open sandwich, Danish style, rather than two pieces of bread, might be the small difference that leads to a longer term healthy weight. Eating fewer potatoes at night, rather than cutting them out entirely, might be all the change that we need.

Carbohydrates are an important part of a healthy diet. They provide energy, fibre, vitamins and minerals. They also, as we'll see later, work well for our gut bacteria. However, it's also true that too many carbs can lead to us putting on weight. And too many processed carbs lead to that, and an urge to eat more.

The reality may be complicated. But we're intelligent animals - we can work our way through it.

Crazy diets: William Banting

William Banting was a nice enough chap, born in 1796. He was an undertaker by trade but is much better known for being the first person to popularise a diet.

He was, for a while, quite a portly fellow. It made his job more challenging, so he went to his doctor who advised a strict regime. He ate four meals a day, consisting of meat, vegetables, fruit, and quite a considerable quantity of wine, sherry and madeira. (Echoes of the old William the Conqueror regime we'll come to later...)

He was so thrilled with his success that he published a pamphlet, and in a piece of advice that I particularly love he writes: "The dry toast or rusk may have a tablespoonful of spirit to soften it, which will prove acceptable." Nothing like a bit of whisky or gin on your dry toast to help it slip down more easily...

He avoided sugar, potatoes, starch, beer, milk and butter (beer is banned, but gin on your toast is fine - I'm sure there's some logic somewhere). Banting's pamphlet was popular for years, and is probably the model for modern diets. Initially, he published the booklet at his own expense but it was so popular that he was determined to sell it to the general public. The third and later editions were published by Harrison, London.

The popularity of the pamphlet was such that the questions "Do you bant?" or "Are you banting?", became slang for dieting.

Banting's booklet is still available online and a most entertaining read it is too.

Clean eating: Gluten-free, Dairy-free, Fun-free

Maybe you've noticed that almost all of the eating plans remove whole food groups from our diet, and almost all of them lead to over-eating. This is certainly true of all the macronutrients - protein, fat and carbohydrates. But what about gluten, dairy and or the 'nightshade' family (potatoes and tomatoes)? It's terribly fashionable to swear off such things.

A clean eating regime promises that you'll be clean inside and out, all scrubbed and glowing. It intimates that even your life won't be messy. We all hope that soon we'll have our dream body, that we can fit into our skinny jeans, hope we'll feel good on the beach this year. And alongside that, we hope that any other mess in our lives will clear itself up, because we'll feel so calm and 'together'. Somehow, cleaning up our diet, will miraculously clean up everything.

It doesn't matter whether it's our relationships or how we usually medicate ourselves with food, once we're 'clean', we'll deal with it. Our irritability when we're tired will vanish. The fact that we hate getting up at 6am to exercise will disappear. Our inability to resist desserts, will be replaced with a zen-like countenance, a lack of interest in sugar and a monk-like reserve of patience that means we never argue with our loved ones again. How disappointed I have been to find myself still whacking the snooze button, unable to haul my sorry self out of bed, just as grumpy as ever. In fact, dietary deprivation has sometimes made me even grumpier. I suspect I'm not alone in that.

So what does 'clean eating' mean and what does it do? It's a relatively recent term, and at first meant avoiding processed foods. Over time, more and more foods were on the banned list, until it meant living of fruit and vegetables, and, depending on whose diet you're following loads of meat or none at all. A group of, largely young women, claimed that following this diet had cured all kinds of things from immune disorders to cancer (this last one has now been proved to have been a lie and the author has lost a court case for damages). Many people followed these women (or men) and the diets in the hope that the trials, or illnesses that dogged them would also fall away.

Let's put aside those people with coeliac disease, where eating gluten more or less leads to their bowels dissolving, and focus on the majority of us who don't have a diagnosed complaint. Instead, maybe we feel a bit bloated after a sandwich, or a bit sluggish after a yoghurt smoothie.

The fact of the matter is that 'allergies' are very rare. You'd know if you had one - it's either hives all over your skin or anaphylactic shock, your airways close up and unless someone is on standby with an epi-pen, your future doesn't look good. (Incidentally, they are now able to reverse even the most severe peanut allergies, with minute and increasing exposure to peanuts).

A more sobering truth for many of us is that a small amount of the gluten or dairy leaves us feeling fine. Half a piece of toast. A tablespoon of yoghurt. We don't feel bloated and lethargic after that. This leads to a very unpalatable conclusion. What if we are just eating too much of these things? What if our serving sizes and our meals have become too large? It's not gluten or dairy per-se that's the problem, it's that we have a massive smoothie on top of our meal, or we eat a bowl of pasta that's the equivalent of three or four servings. That's a much more unpleasant truth to face.

When we cut out major food groups, what they are replaced with is often worse than the original. Gluten-free products are usually more processed, higher calorie and lower fibre than the full-gluten alternative. When the European Society for Paediatric Gastroenterology Hepatology and Nutrition compared 654 products to similar items containing gluten, it found that the gluten-free versions had a significantly higher fat content and were often less nutritious than their ordinary equivalents.

Dairy-free products are also chock-full of ingredients that I've never heard of, and there's no evidence that things like soy are better for us. Sugar replacements, we've covered - they're so similar to the real thing, that it's almost pointless swapping.

What I'm voting for, is evaluating how your body feels. If you feel rotten after bread, do all foods containing wheat affect you? Or does it depend on the quantity? Or is it the highly processed stuff? In some instances, perhaps it is you that has changed?

As we get older, some of us experience a change in the amount of lactase we produce - this is what helps us digest dairy products. This means that something we used to eat without a problem when we were younger, may now not be so comfortable. In fact, science shows that 65 percent of the world's population is lactose intolerant. It's particularly prevalent in some races - those that culturally don't usually consume milk, showing that our bodies adapt to our diets.

On the other hand, scientists have looked into gluten sensitivity, and found that it might not be what it seems. (I'm not talking Coeliacs here - that's a different story). They gave gluten-intolerant participants a small sachet of powder to sprinkle on their food. Only a small handful (8 percent in one study, 13 percent in another) were able to tell which weeks they had consumed gluten because they had symptoms. Half the people couldn't tell the difference and the remainder guessed wrong. This means that around 90 percent of the gluten-intolerant participants didn't have a reaction to gluten.

Further investigation showed that some of those who believed that they were gluten intolerant, found their symptoms abated if they followed a FODmap diet.

FODmaps are a group of carbohydrates that are fermented by bacteria in the bowel and can cause symptoms for some individuals. Other research is pointing the finger at pesticides and environmental toxins rather than gluten. In America, crops of wheat are sometimes sprayed with Glyphosate (a weedkiller and poison) to kill the plants to make them easier to harvest. This remains in the wheat, which we then ingest.

My point isn't to catalogue an exhaustive list of intolerances, but rather to show that it can be very tricky to get to the bottom (excuse the pun) of what is actually causing the problem, if you have one. The obvious candidate, such as gluten, isn't always the culprit.

Did you know that tomatoes were considered poisonous in England until very recently. It's only really in the last hundred years that people have been prepared to eat them. And before we conclude that this was another ridiculous food fad, a new theory is that the common use of pewter plates might have been the issue. Pewter reacts with the acid in tomatoes to release lead. So there may indeed have been instances of poisoning. Hard indeed, to accurately pinpoint the culprit.

It's entirely up to you what you enjoy and what suits you. You don't have to sign up for 'clean eating' or renounce dairy forever. You can decide not to eat wheat at every meal. (Actually, it's a good thing to vary your foods - and if you're having cereal for breakfast, sandwiches for lunch and pizza for dinner, effectively wheat three times a day, you might want to introduce some variety. It's good for our bodies to have different foods as they need to source all of the vitamins and minerals.)

You might have a dairy free day a week, or skip it in your coffee. The point is that you're in charge. You get to decide, based on what suits you and what you like.

Imagine that. It's almost treating ourselves like adults...

ACTION

Notice how your body feels. Do you have intestinal issues after specific foods? If so, is it just bloating, or do you have more unpleasant symptoms?

Does cutting down on quantity help, or do you feel better if you eliminate them entirely?

Experiment with different foods and notice what makes you feel good.

Because I'm not getting enough sleep

Remember those days when we used go out all night, and then sit down to a massive fry up? Exhausted but wired from dancing or drinking until dawn, we'd collapse laughing in a cafe, stomachs rumbling at the prospect of a large plate of eggs, bacon and toast slathered in butter. It might seem like a while ago now, but there was a reason why those fry-ups tasted so good. Lack of sleep can make you really hungry.

The sad truth is that some of us feel exhausted yet wired most days, and not because we've been out to a good old party but because our kids kept us up all night or we had an international work phone call late in the evening, or we had to get up early to get the household organised. We're on an endless treadmill of tiredness, stumbling from one thing to the next, without the the joys of the night before.

There are times we eat when we're not hungry, just in order to pep ourselves up and keep ourselves going. It might be late afternoon, you have another meeting at work, and you eat a snack, not because you are particularly hungry, but because you're getting tired, and need a boost.

Stephanie, a nurse, would come home exhausted from a long shift at the hospital, rush to the kitchen and eat several pieces of toast and butter before soldiering on to prepare a meal and tidy the house. She felt helpless eating the toast, unable to function without it, yet knowing it was a bad idea when she was cooking a meal that would be ready in less than an hour.

Tiredness isn't usually a sign that we need sometimes to eat, what it usually means is that we need a rest. But resting is deeply uncool these days. (actually, I suspect the phrase 'deeply uncool' is also uncool.) It's very fashionable to be so busy that you don't have time to rest, time to eat, time for yourself. We're all running from one thing to the next - to build in some 'down time' is tantamount to saying that your life is empty.

To actually admit that you took a twenty minute nap or lie-down is almost akin to admitting that you voted for Trump. People will gasp and step away from you in horror. There will be whispers at the school gate.

Too little sleep may bring on a form of the marijuana "munchies", according to a recent study that found sleep-deprived people craved crisps, sweets and biscuits far more than healthier foods. Skimping on sleep appears to alter brain chemicals in much the same way as the hunger-boosting ingredient in cannabis.

Fourteen men and women spent two four-day sessions at the Chicago University's clinical research centre. The volunteers' time in bed was controlled, so that on one visit they averaged 7.5 hours of sleep a night, but on the other only four hours 11 minutes a night. During their stays, the volunteers ate identical meals, dished out at 9am, 2pm and 7pm.

After the fourth night of each study, the participants were offered a range of snacks. The sleep-deprived felt a strong urge to binge on fatty foods, and this was most intense in the late afternoon and early evening, when snacking is most linked to weight gain. They avidly consumed high-fat snacks even when they had eaten a solid meal containing 90 percent of their recommended daily calories only two hours earlier. Typically, the sleepy participants ate 300 calories in snacks, far more than they needed to make up for their extra hours awake.

The scientists looked at various substances in the volunteers' blood, including chemicals called endocannabinoids. They found that when sleep-deprived, volunteers had higher and more persistent levels of endocannabinoid 2-AG, a chemical that ramps up the pleasure felt when eating, especially sweet or salty high-fat foods. "We know that marijuana activates the endocannabinoid system and causes people to overeat when they are not hungry, and they normally eat yummy sweet and fatty foods," Hanlon said. "Sleep restriction may cause overeating by acting in the same manner."

While there is still much to be understood about how lack of sleep affects appetite, perhaps one of the best techniques to help us lose weight and stop cheating on ourselves, is more sleep?

We worked together on solutions for Stephanie and she agreed that the family could eat fifteen minutes later, and she could have fifteen minutes to herself: just lying down if she chose, or reading or meditating.

This took the pressure off her, allowed herself a bit of time to recover without eating.

Of course, you don't have to admit that you had a rest. You don't want to become a social pariah. Just sneak in a nap or two, instead of sneaking the food, and see what happens.

When people ask how you miraculously dropped the pounds, you can just answer that they'd be so shocked to know the truth that you couldn't possibly tell them.

I'm stressed: that's why I'm fat in the first place...

Stress and weight control are mutually exclusive. Biologically, they don't work well together. When you are stressed, your body will do everything it can to hold onto weight. Stress raises the level of cortisol in the body, which increases fat storage, particularly around the abdomen. Stress also reduces insulin efficiency, which means that you crave more sugar, and more sugar is converted to fat. This means that the very presence of stress will make it harder for you to manage your weight, just due to your biological programming.

That's cheered us all up then, hasn't it?

Stress can also lead to mindless eating.... Walking in from a stressful day at the office and browsing the cupboards for something tasty to eat – a handful of nuts perhaps, a spoonful of ice cream out of the tub, a biscuit, perhaps a just a smidge of chocolate. And before you know it, you've eaten more than a meal's worth without noticing.

Or perhaps it is driving home – stopping for petrol, and just buying a treat to take home that never quite makes it home. And then there's eating at your desk – grinding through the day chocolate by chocolate, muffin by biscuit, just to get to home time. Until you lose track of everything you've consumed, because you haven't tasted or remembered even half of it.

These are coping mechanisms for the stressful and fast-paced world that we live in. Fairly obviously, they are coping mechanisms that make it worse for us. They make it worse by increasing stress. When you wake in the morning the first stress of the day is finding that the waistband of your clothes is too tight. Or knowing that you don't look or feel your best, because of the mindless eating.

This behaviour has been replicated time and again in laboratories all over the world. Scientists investigate the effect of acute and psychological stress on food intake, examining how much participants eat in the absence of hunger, for both normal and overweight men and women. Energy intake from sweet foods was significantly higher in the stress condition than in the control. To quote: "We conclude that acute psychological stress is associated with eating in the absence of hunger, especially in vulnerable individuals characterized by disinhibited eating behavior and sensitivity to chronic stress."

What this means is that not only do we eat more when stressed, but that we make ourselves more vulnerable to this by dieting, which 'disinhibits' eating behaviour.

Realistically, we're never going to get rid of stress. There's even evidence that some stress is good for us - it gees us up, and gets us going. It's just how we cope with it, especially in a world where we seem to have less and less time. (See previous section).

If we know that we tend to eat more when we are stressed, and we know that eating more can then add to our load, with worries about weight gain and health, then how do we break the cycle?

This is when it helps to come back to hunger and satisfaction. Return to how your body feels and see whether it's hungry. Notice whether the food makes you feel less stressed or more. There is a certain oblivion that large quantities of carbohydrate can offer, a zoned-out, stuffed-to-the-gunnels, sedated lethargy, that fades the stresses to a more distant hum. At least, until the guilt sets in.

If you find that you want that zoned out feeling in the evening, work out if you can achieve that state with foods that are less hard on the body that processed carbohydrates. Would a large bowl of pumpkin soup with whole meal bread do the same? Perhaps a yoga class might help soothe the parts of you that are wrecked by stress?

There is a great deal of evidence that fresh air and walking is very therapeutic in such instances. The problem is that we'd all rather collapse on the sofa in front of a box-set with a large supply of comfort food.

We'll move onto how food can act like a drug - so it's natural for us to use it like one. And like drugs, its worth remembering the side effects. Do you really feel better in that state of oblivion? Or do you just feel numb and dead to the world?

If you're feeling stressed, try and take the time to look after yourself with healing foods and more rest. Be gentle. Ask for help if you need it.

There might be a different way to the old habits. The question is, are you brave enough to explore it?

We use food for comfort.

"Oh, my boss has cancelled my review, that's why I'm eating".

"I've put on weight, so I may as well have the whole packet of biscuits".

"I need ice cream straight from the tub because my boyfriend dumped me."

Eating has become the drug we use to medicate ourselves in an increasingly fast-paced and hostile world. When we are stressed, or lonely, or upset, or just can't deal with it any more, where else can we turn but food?

What comfort we gain from the warm, greasy crunch of chips, or the soothing melting sweetness of chocolate. What solace there is in the creamy richness of a large tub of ice cream. What bliss in the sugary crunch of cookies....

There are many reasons why eating is comforting. In evolutionary terms, if you're eating, you aren't starving, which is definitely a plus. It also means you're not being chased by a large wild animal, but must be safe in your cave. In biological terms, the very act of eating releases a number of hormones and chemicals that soothe and calm us. It is absolutely possible to feel drunk or high on food alone.

There are wonderful associations with, and reminders of, celebrations and family meals that give us comfort and solace. It's because of these, and many more emotional connections, we forget that food is there to feed us when we are hungry, not when we are emotionally empty.

One of the most important things we can learn, is how to nourish and care for ourselves emotionally, without using food, or drugs. If we can comfort ourselves without resorting to food, we are much freer to choose when we eat something. We can eat it because we'd really enjoy it at that moment, not because without it, life looks pretty damn bleak.

I don't think it much matters which emotional triggers drive you to eat - whether it's anger or sorrow. I don't think it matters what you use to comfort yourself when you feel rubbish. The only thing that matters is finding a way to take better care of yourself.

To this end, make some time, and sit down, and try to imagine that you've been given an unlimited budget to employ someone whose sole role is to make you happy. They will do nothing for anyone else. Their sole focus is you. Their only reason for being is to look after you, and do whatever you need to make your life better and happier. Try to write a job description for someone whose only role in life is to look after you. What would you have them do? Bring you a cup of tea in bed? Lay out your clothes for you? Drive you to work? Cook you dinner? Tidy your house? They are on call to you all day every day and their only purpose is to make you happy.

Write down every single thing they would do for you. Work through the day and think what you need at every moment. Consider what they would say to you - would they encourage you to go for a walk? Would they praise your efforts for the day? Try to envisage this in as much detail as you can.

If you think I'm going to suggest you present this to your husband or boyfriend with an ultimatum... dream on (I wish!). This is what you need to do for yourself.

The job description you have written, is your own. This is what you can do for yourself, to look after yourself, to keep yourself safe. Make your bed, if that soothes you when you get home. Keep the house tidier if that reduces your stress levels. Stop calling your mother if that drives you to the biscuit tin. You won't go to hell. You don't have to do all of it - just start with the bits that will make a difference to how you feel, and how you cope with life.

It takes time to learn how to care for ourselves, especially if we're running a household and looking after a family. We are too often last. But just like the aeroplanes, where you fit your own oxygen mask before helping others, sometimes you have to show compassion to yourself in order to be there for everyone else.

Another thing to consider, as you reach for your comfort food, is the Diminishing Law of Marginal Utility. I know - catchy title, right? Basically, this means that the first bite of anything is usually the most delicious.

Each successive bite is progressively less delicious as the craving is satisfied. This is Economic theory, not Psychology.

The first mouthful is what we've been waiting for - we taste it and our bodies and brains fire up. The next mouthful we notice less, until eventually we are eating on autopilot.

This works until the final mouthful, which is almost as delicious as the first. Perhaps as the brain registers that the experience is almost over.

Is this true for you? What about just having two bites: the first and the last, and leave the rest of the cake or whatever it is. Would that be enough?

ACTION

Write that job description.

Consider Economic Theory and whether it rings true for you. Is the first bite really the most satisfying? Try experimenting and seeing which mouthful is the most delicious for you.

Fasting. That's the whole reason.

Fasting has been a fashionable thing to do, on and off, throughout history. It's going through a renaissance at the moment, championed by the likes of Gwyneth Paltrow on her blog 'Goop'. Fasting means going without food (or without food and water) for a period, generally of more than one day. Its origins are religious where it was believed abstaining from eating purified either the priest or the sacrificial victim for ceremonies and rituals, often involved the death of the purified one.

Today, the ceremonies most likely to engender this behaviour are The Oscars, weddings or bikini holidays: a far cry from sanctified and holy services of old. Although maybe not - the Aztecs has some pretty wild rituals. Nonetheless, the sense of being somehow 'purified' through fasting hasn't died out. We are led to believe that there is something morally superior about those who can go without food, something elevated. Something special.

Fasting advocates speak of feeling cleaner, lighter, of mental clarity. For most of us, (or at least me) who might describe ourselves as sluggish, unkempt and forgetful, this appears to be some pinnacle of existence. Could I really undergo a such a radical transformation just by eliminating food?

Fasting can also be one of the quickest ways to really mess up your body. New research on the neurobiology of eating is showing this. Our appetite and eating is governed largely by two systems in the brain. The first is kind of the like the system that controls our temperature – it is a homeostatic set of mechanisms which make us feel hungry and full in response to our body's needs. The hormone leptin controls this. If prolonged dieting results in weight loss, the amount of leptin secreted will be reduced, making us more hungry.

However, scientists have found that the reduction in leptin levels with ongoing fasting is disproportionate to the reduction in adipose mass. This means, that fasting makes your leptin plummet, even if you're not losing weight, or not losing much. They conclude that 'the ability of fasting to deactivate this presumed physiological satiety system may have been advantageous in environments characterized by rapid changes in food availability.' Either way, fasting 'deactivates' the system that makes us feel full. And we really don't want to do that.

The second is a hedonic (or pleasure-based) mechanism that makes us desire food and feel pleasure when eating. In this system, the 'wanting' of food is moderated by the homeostatic system to a degree. I'll talk about how this gets out of whack later.

If you fast for a long time and essential nutrients such as protein are lacking from your diet, an intense urge to eat occurs as a result of our homeostatic system. This is wired to ensure our survival so that we don't starve to death.

If after a period of food restriction, people are exposed to 'highly palatable' (delicious, to you or me) food, they over eat in response to that urge and the tendency to over consume or binge when exposed to these foods remains for several months afterwards. Underpinning these longer term changes in the brain is an imbalance in the chemical transmitters involved in the hedonistic system.

Did you read that? Several months afterwards...

Research is showing that dieting interspersed with intermittent consumption of snacks and other highly palatable food might lead to permanent changes in the hedonic mechanism of eating.

Permanent changes...If you fast, you may forever mess up your eating mechanism.

To be fair, there seem to be benefits to fasting - the immune system kicks in and repairs the body. New research, that has been well publicised with the 5:2 diet is showing that there may be health benefits to it. It's just that for many of us, the price it too high - we do rebound eating that undoes all the good. If you're a cheater, it maybe a step too far.

If you're fasting to lose weight, it's not an efficient way to do that. The lack of nutrients mean that its very easy to lose muscle as well as fat, and we want to hold onto muscle as much as possible. We'll see later that as we age, our muscle decreases, and this is the part of our body that burns most calories (aside from the brain), so it's in our interests to preserve it.

Let's address some other issues. Fasting doesn't purify your body. You body is constantly purifying itself: your kidneys are flushing out excess proteins and toxins and expelling them in urine. Your skin is also getting rid of unwanted elements through sweat. The digestive system and liver are constantly working to 'purify' your body. They need no particular help to do this. This is their function.

If you are suffering from a severe condition such as cirrhosis of the liver, then you may wish to consider lightening up on your body (less alcohol perhaps?) but otherwise, most of us live in clean, healthy environments where our bodies can cope with the day to day demands placed on them.

As for achieving mental clarity and feeling clean and light? For shaking off the torpor and sluggishness that dogs us all?

Perhaps I'm forever destined to get to the top of the stairs and wonder what on earth I was supposed to be doing or getting.

My gut bacteria told me to...

Did you know you have one hundred trillion bacteria in your gut? That's more than the total number of cells in your body, and each one has it's own genetic code and everything! (well, not everything, they don't have shoes, for example).

They only weigh a couple of kilograms in total, so sadly we can't blame them for the number on the scale. However, we could possibly blame them for something else... our cheating.

Whilst we've known about these chaps for a while, it's only very recently that their role in our mood and choices have become apparent.

Your microbiome (this is the term for all those bacteria) are altered and changed by what you eat, because what you eat changes their environment and different ones thrive. Scientists have found different profiles of bacteria according to whether community lives in Africa eating nuts, or in the Arctic eating seal meat. The bacteria change according to whether you're consuming large quantities of fast foods, or whether you're a vegan.

As scientists learn more, these bacteria appear to play an important role in our immune systems, our health and even our mood.

New research shows that they could influence when you feel hunger cravings and what you're hungry for. It's already proven that what we eat changes the bacteria in our stomach. Now scientists think that the little critters actually pipe up with a menu request.

In the past few years, scientists have suggested that the bacteria in our gut might be able to influence not only our appetite, but also what we fancy eating. The bacteria send messages up the Vagus nerve to the brain. It's too early to say whether they are the ones demanding pastries rather than salad, but it's a possibility.

According to Schwarz and Sclafani, the gut is a highly complex nervous system. It is the body's "second brain", and this second brain becomes conditioned to wanting more sugar, sending messages back to the 'actual' brain that are very hard to fight.

There is also evidence that they become used to being fed at certain times. If you usually have a snack at 4pm, and decide to skip it, in order to lose a bit of weight, your gut bacteria may have other ideas...

On the other hand, while gut bacteria aren't going to lose your weight for you, they can certainly help. They influence us and our appetites, but we can actually control them. We could kill them all off with a dose of antibiotics, which further depletes our immune systems. This is a strong argument for avoiding antibiotics unless we really needs them - using them when we have a cold makes it even harder for our systems to recover.

We can also change what we eat as the things that we consume determine what kinds of bacteria we have. Most of us know that yoghurt is full of 'good' bacteria that helps the populations that live in our intestines. There are lots of other foods that also work similarly, largely fermented foods such as sauerkraut and miso. Most fruits and vegetables also generate good bacteria that work in our favour.

The bottom line is that our bacteria, whilst they number many many trillion, can only influence our decisions. Certain bacteria may mean that we're more likely to cheat. But we are the ones who get the final say what we eat. And we also get to decide whether we feed the nice bacteria, or the nasty ones. Needless to say, the nasty ones always want sugar.

Why couldn't it be the other way round, for once?

Summary

Managing our hunger and not eating more than we choose to is far easier when we are working in sync with our bodies. It's very easy to get out of whack, especially in our fast-paced world, full of sugary treats.

Maintaining a consistent blood sugar level is the key to this, which means avoiding insulin highs and lows. Trying to eat low glycemic, or at least avoid massive sugar hits will help, as will eating protein with every meal. Sugar substitutes don't really help with this at all - you may as well have the real thing.

Try to have a bit of everything in your diet - some fat, some carbs and some protein. We don't need to cut out any of these to lose weight or be healthy, and in fact, removing any one of these tends to cause a massive backlash as our systems drive us to eat it - and cheat. In fact, you don't need to cut out any food groups at all.

Fasting, although it may help our bodies repair themselves, is very hard to manage without our blood sugar levels rocketing all over the place and our energy levels struggling. All of this leads to more overeating once the fast is over, or, if it's really bad, half way through our intended abstinence.

If you're interested in it, look into cultivating good gut bacteria. Lots of fruit and vegetables help, as does avoiding antibiotics.

Make sure you get enough sleep, and rest when you're tired rather than eat to keep yourself going a bit longer. Look after yourself. We each only get one body, and we do tend to expect a lot of them.

CHAPTER FOUR
PSYCHOLOGY AND NEUROSCIENCE

Not only can we set up our bodies to work against us, but our brains can do the same.

We might think that we are in charge, that we know why we do what we do, and are in control of our actions. But a more likely model is that our brains have 'programs' that they run, to save energy and to allow us to concentrate on something else.

Food manufacturers have cottoned on to how they can play these subconscious programs to have us eat more than ever we realise.

It's amazing how our brains work! Let's find out how to stop them being hacked by sugar and fat.

How did the packet end up empty?

Have you ever driven home from work, pulled into your driveway, and realised that you have absolutely no memory whatsoever of the journey? Perhaps you commute to work, and you find yourself at your desk, with minimal or no recollection of the various trains or buses you took.

When behaviours become habitual, or regular, our brains relegate them to the subconscious. We don't need to focus on them, so the brain switches our consciousness to focus on something else: our phone, our worries, our plans.

Unfortunately, this same mechanism can come into play when we have regular eating habits or addictions.

The brain is used to us thinking: "Hmm, that was a stressful day. I really could use some … (insert 'comfort food of choice')…" And it knows exactly how to get us to the shop to buy some, and get the food into our bags and then into our mouths.

Many people have told me that they have believed that they were sticking rigorously to their diet, only to find themselves sitting on their couch with an empty food packet on their lap, and no idea of how it happened.

One of my first clients was a Mum called Maureen. She would insist that she ate without realising it. "I opened the packet, it was a packet of granola. I buy it for my kids, I don't eat it, it's too fattening. But I just wanted one of those banana chips, so I opened it to find one of those. There was one at the top, and I ate it. I recall delving back into the bag for a particularly large clump with a sultana in it. And the next thing I knew, fifteen minutes or more had passed, and the bag was half empty. I honestly don't remember doing it!"

The brain has well-worn paths. It is used to a flood of sugar at certain points in the day, and can turn off your consciousness while your preprogrammed behaviour runs, acquiring the substance, and then ingesting it, all without realising it.

I have, in the past, sworn off sugar, only to have a friend point out the chocolate I was shovelling into my mouth from the bowl on her table. It was in front of me, and my hand reached for it, bypassing all my declarations that I was never going to eat it again. A tad embarrassing.

Not only is this embarrassing. It's extraordinary. It seems that our left hand literally doesn't know what the right hand is doing.

The first thing to do, is not to add to your woes with a large helping of guilt. These are well worn paths that you are travelling. Part of your being is just doing what it thinks you want.

David Kessler, the former head of the US government's most powerful food agency, the FDA, talks of 'priming'. Sometimes just one taste of a food, a single bite, is enough to trigger conditioned 'hyper-eating'. Priming involves stimulating areas of your brain. The use of the word 'conditioned' means it's already a habit. Your body recognises the primer, or taste, as the beginning of a conditioned or habituated pattern of behaviour.

The problem is that it's hard to shut those habits off. Once primed, they stay activated and you may continue to eat until all the food is gone. That's what the food industry knows when it tells us "Bet you can't eat just one."

The good news is that priming only holds power for a short time. If you eat one piece of candy and there's a bowl of them in front of you, chances are you will keep eating more. But if no more are available or you have to search for them, the priming response may be undermined.

If you travel these paths less, or stop doing the behaviour, the priming will fade and it will stop being automatic, and you will not feel so compelled. But how to get there?

It's easiest to stop the habit in the earliest stages. If you know there are times when you eat unconsciously, and they are usually in a certain place, or preceded by a certain thing, then try to address the first step.

If you can eat an entire packet of biscuits in front of the television, either don't have the biscuits in the house, or put something on the couch, to remind you that if you are going to eat biscuits, that you have decided that you are going to eat them at the table, with full focus on them and full enjoyment.

ACTION

Your brain may hijack your best intentions. How can you support your decisions to change a habit or stop mindless eating? List some ways that you can break the habit once it starts without you realising. What things can you put in place to remind you of what is happening?

Food's reward is immediate, weight loss is slow

Back in the 1970's, another psychology experiment was taking place, using marshmallows. Small children were sat, one by one, in a room with a marshmallow. They were told that if they could resist eating it for fifteen minutes, they would be rewarded with an additional marshmallow. Being able to hold off is apparently a good predictor of future life success. I sometimes wonder how a starving person on a detox regime would fare in the this experiment. I can imagine them cramming the marshmallow into their mouths and then running riot through the laboratory, ransacking cupboards, determined to seek out the mother load - the whole packet.

Behavioural psychology has a lot to say about reward. All of it shows that if a behaviour is rewarded, we repeat it. We know this intuitively, and use it when rearing our children, training our pets, incentivising our employees.

With weight loss, this doesn't really work. The reward for eating a cream cake is immediate. It's delicious, the craving is satisfied. We associate pleasant feelings and memories with the cream cake. Our weight doesn't change that day. There are no repercussions.

If we eat a salad, we aren't rewarded with instant slimness. In fact, we have to persist with healthier behaviours for some time in order for the results to show.

Which means that for dieting, all of the reward mechanisms are messed up. We experience a 'reward' for the fattening foods, the forbidden ones, which trigger the hedonic response (mentioned earlier) which is one of the most powerful rewards there is. But we don't see our belt suddenly loosening with a mouthful of vegetables.

James tells me:

"Look, I dieted for four days. I gave up pies for lunch, suffered loads of crap from the guys, told I was being a big girl's blouse for eating a salad sandwich. I didn't go out for beers with them, and four days later, my gut is still as big.

I may as well give in and have a few pints on a Friday."

It takes a lot to trust that new behaviours will deliver in the long run. And sometimes the instant reward is more gratifying.

So we cheat.

We say: 'I've been good, so I deserve it.' Or 'Look at everything I do for everyone else: I need a little something for myself.' Or 'I've had salad all week, so I'll have chocolate on the weekend.'

Our psychology means we are drawn to tempting short-term options. We may "know" about the long-term dangers or benefits, but they do not exert much force on our current decisions. This has been proven in many experiments involving financial decisions, health and more. It's being proved on a larger scale with how we are treating our planet.

Detoxes, diets and eating plans fall into the short term category for several reasons. Firstly, by their very nature, they are short term activities with a start and end date. We don't plan (usually) to continue them indefinitely. Secondly, we are faced daily with the decision to either stick to the eating plan and gain a longer term yet vague outcome, or 'cheat' and eat something delicious and naughty right now.

The doughnut in your hand is far more concrete than the promise of weight loss in a month's time, especially if you've failed at weight loss before. So you take the doughnut. Which brings us back to the marshmallows. Can we wait for a better reward?

But there's more to it than the reward aspect, there is our view of what we'll do for a little while, and what we're prepared to accept forever. Because we view dieting or eating plans as a short term activity, we include in them behaviours that we could never sustain in the long term. These behaviours might include never eating carbs after 6pm, or swearing off all sugar. A good question to ask, with any new eating behaviour is: Can I do this for the rest of my life?

If the answer is no, then why do it for three weeks? Once the three weeks is up, you'll stop the eating plan and return to your old behaviour, and, lo and behold, with the old behaviour will come all the weight. you put on weight that way last time, you'll put on weight that way again.

How about considering which behaviours you can sustain indefinitely?

I couldn't swear off cheese forever. But I can ask myself each meal whether or not I really want it. I can have it if I do, but if not, I'll wait until the next meal. It sounds simple and unlikely to work, but it's amazing how giving yourself permission to have something, takes some of its allure away. Why not wait until you really want it, and have it then?

You may ask yourself whether it's worth building rewards into your diet, such as rewarding yourself with a massage for every week that you stick to it. The problem with this is that extrinsic rewards have been shown to damage motivation. Paying children to draw greatly reduced their enjoyment of it, until they only wanted to do it when monetary reward was on the table. Until then the drawing had been rewards enough in itself.

Somehow, we have to find a way to eat that is reward in itself. This isn't going to happen through deprivation. Neither is it going to happen with a diet that leads to weight gain, low energy and worse health. It's harder to work it out for ourselves - how much we want to eat and of what, versus the pay-offs in terms of how we feel.

ACTION

Try to weigh up the short term pleasures of foods versus the longer term benefits (whether health or weight loss) that you are pursuing. Does that alter how much you want to eat something?

If you are going to change a behaviour, or give something up, make sure it's something you can sustain for the rest of your life. Ask yourself if you're really committed to it.

Why you want more: what the food manufacturers don't want you to know.

I am working at my computer, half concentrating on what I'm writing and half thinking about chocolate. Creamy, smooth milk chocolate. Then I think that I might rather have it with some crunch - rice bubbles or biscuit. Saliva rushes into my mouth and I find myself in the kitchen, ransacking the cupboards.

I break off a piece of chocolate, and it melts on my tongue, sweet and smooth before I bite down on the fragile crispness inside. It's divine. I've had a piece, addressed my craving.

So why do I now want more? And why do I want it more urgently than I wanted the first piece?

If I ate an apple, the thought of eating a second would be faintly repulsive. One is enough. So why isn't that the case with chocolate, or biscuits, or crisps, ice cream....

Having spent much of my career in marketing for the global chocolate, biscuit and ice cream brands (you already know how good that was for my weight) I can answer that. When developing a new product, many different iterations are created and then tested, repeatedly, through focus groups and research. One of the key questions is:

"Once you have eaten one, do you want the next one more, or less?"

For unprocessed foods (fruits, vegetables) once you have eaten one, you want the next one slightly less. You feel full, or at least satisfied with that flavour. To eat more of it feels boring, nauseating, uncomfortable or all three.

For processed foods, the aim is to make the consumer want the next one more than the first. Of course. This means that we eat more, buy more, and the manufacturer makes more money.

For us to eat more, the product needs a combination of elements. Firstly, it mustn't be too filling. So fibre is removed and particles ground down to tiny fragments so that our digestive systems don't register it. This also means that the food has a highly palatable feel in the mouth.

Often it vanishes with almost no chewing, dissolves. This adds to the sense that we haven't eaten, and is also highly pleasurable. Perhaps it reminds us of our first taste of milk that needed no work to chew.

Secondly, the food must trigger the hedonic response. This is the pleasure centre in our brains. It responds to such things as heroin, cocaine, sugar, fat and even salt... lighting up like a beacon and sending waves of happiness and delight through our bodies.

New research is showing that over time our brains actually become addicted to the natural opioids that are triggered by sugar and fat consumption. Much like the classic drugs of abuse such as cocaine, alcohol and nicotine, a diet loaded with sugar can generate excessive reward signals in the brain which can override one's self-control and lead to addiction.

One study out of France, showed that rats addicted to cocaine, switched to sweetened water when given the choice between that and water with cocaine. The rats preferred to press the button that delivered a drink of sugary syrup than the button which injected them with cocaine. They choose sugar over the drug to which they're addicted, finding intense sweetness more rewarding to the brain than cocaine. So if tiny little mice are opting for sugar over hard drugs, there may be reasons why we also turn to it to ease our passage through life.

There are strict laws around what can be put in pharmaceutical drugs. But the same legislation has not been applied to what can be added to foodstuffs. If something originates from a plant that we usually eat, then it can be processed in any manner and still regarded as edible.

This strikes me as extraordinary, given that some of our most potent drugs come from plants. Heroin comes from the poppy, and we eat poppy seeds in cakes. (Apparently, if you eat a large quantity of them, you can get a faint high... I haven't tried this.) Cocaine comes from the Coca leaf.

High fructose corn syrup come from sweetcorn, and may act on the body like a drug, but this has not been considered even though the degree and nature of processing is similar to class A drugs. Certainly, our bodies no longer recognise it as a food - there are no feelings of satiation or fullness, there are no vitamins, minerals or other benefits to the body and it creates cravings.

The hedonic response can be most strongly generated through a combination of sugar, fat and salt. If you add salt to sugar, things taste less sweet, which means that sugar can be used in ever larger quantities, without the product tasting too sugary. Of course, this sends our bodies into overdrive.

The fact that you want more is not because there is something wrong with you. Your body is working exactly as it should. You want more because there is something amiss with what we are eating. Your brain is lighting up like a beacon and every system in your body is being played to make you want more.

I'm not saying don't eat these things. I eat them. I enjoy them, and one of the reasons that I enjoy them is because they provoke this great wave of pleasure.

However, when I eat food that are highly processed or very sweet, I acknowledge that there is a drug-like effect, and that I could easily eat more. Just as I choose not to inject heroin, I choose not to eat more and more. Now that my body and I work together on these things, the food doesn't control me. I am in charge of what goes into my mouth.

All of this is easier, if you follow some of the other pointers in the other chapters.

Neuroscience is catching up with food manufacturers

Until recently, research focused on physical hunger, and assumed that being obese meant you were just incredibly hungry and therefore had to eat loads. I suspect a number of us could have told them that eating dessert has nothing to do with feeling hungry or full. And at last, research is catching up.

Michael Lowe, a clinical psychologist at Drexel University coined the term "hedonic hunger" in 2007. He says: "A lot of overeating, maybe all of the eating people do beyond their energy needs, is based on consuming some of our most palatable foods." No kidding! Please don't tell me it took years of scientific research to work that out. Who gets fat on cucumber?

Research shows that extremely sweet or fatty foods light up the brain's reward circuit in the same way that cocaine, drugs, gambling and other 'addictive' behaviours do. The brain begins to react to fatty and sugary foods even before they enter our mouth: just seeing them excites the reward circuit. As soon as such it touches the tongue, taste buds send signals to the brain, which ramps up dopamine. The result is an intense feeling of pleasure.

Over time, the brain gets desensitised, so to get the same 'high' or pleasurable feeling, we need to eat more. It's the same with any addiction. We need a bigger and bigger hit. The brain needs a lot more sugar and fat to reach the same level of pleasure that it once felt with smaller amounts of the foods.

This isn't a sign of us being weak. It's us being in thrall to an addictive circuit in our brain. When dopamine levels drop, we feel down. So no wonder we turn to fat and sugar. They are literally acting as an anti-depressant. Food is acting like a drug.

Way back in 1976, Professor Anthony Sclafani was studying appetite and weight gain, when he noticed something strange about his lab rats. When they ate rat food, they put on weight normally. But when they ate processed food from a supermarket, they ballooned in a matter of days. Their appetite for sugary foods was insatiable: they just carried on eating.

When he gave his rats access to a variety of palatable human foods, as well as standard rodent chow, the rats completely ignored the chow, closing to gorge on the palatable food and rapidly becoming obese. Later renamed the 'cafeteria diet', it remains the most rapid and effective way of producing dietary obesity and metabolic syndrome in rodents using solid food.

The more processed it is, the more out bodies recognise it as a drug, rather than as food. The satisfaction circuits related to eating and nutrition no longer trigger (there is little fibre to make us feel full, minimal nutrients to sate those needs). Instead, we ingest it as mouthfuls of anti-depressant, needing more and more over time.

David Kessler, the former head of the US government's most powerful food agency, the FDA, and the person responsible for introducing warnings on cigarette packets in the early 90s, believes that sugar, through its metabolisation by the gut and hence the brain, is extremely addictive, just like cigarettes or alcohol. He believes that sugar is hedonic. He says eating it is "highly pleasurable. It gives you this momentary bliss. When you're eating food that is highly hedonic, it sort of takes over your brain."

The good news is that the reward circuits can change back. If you went cold turkey on fat and sugar for a few weeks, it would take a much smaller dose to stimulate those dopamine hits. Of course, after a few small hits, you'd once again need larger ones.

The problem isn't us. It's the food. We are a clever species and we have created foods that are like drugs, sending us into paroxysms of bliss, and leaving us wanting more. This is making the food companies rich, and it's making us fat.

So: what to do? Even though I know this is what is happening to my body, I still don't want to live a life without ice cream, crammed with cookie dough or fudge. I don't want to go to France and resist a buttery, flaky croissant. Sometimes, a moist slice of lemon cake, with a tart yet sugary icing is all that will do.

Belinda, another client, recognised that hedonic eating was a major problem for her. She would follow a sugar-free diet for a while, intuitively knowing that this was her weak spot and would feel better.

"I felt a sense of reclaimed power," she said, "I was the one in control, not the sugar. I felt virtuous and energised. But then something would happen. A birthday cake at work, or a stressful day at work or my son would bring back some home made fudge from school, and I'd just have one mouthful. That's all. just one, thinking I could resist. And then I'd be back on it."

Belinda found a two-fold approach helped. Firstly, once she knew what her neurochemistry was doing, she stopped blaming herself for being weak. This was an important step. "Suddenly, I didn't see myself as disgusting for giving in. I saw myself as human. I saw it as natural, almost, that my body is designed to respond like that. It was enormously freeing. But interestingly, it didn't mean that I felt it was out of my control, in some ways, I saw that it was my decision whether I let that reward pathway take over my life or not. Now I'm very conscious that the more sugar I eat, the more I want, so I keep an eye on it. If I find myself craving it, I work out whether I'm really hungry for it, or whether my brain just wants a quick fix. I also keep a lot less of it in the house. It's just too easy for me to eat."

Belinda decided, that for her, a house full of sugar was something that she would struggle with. In similar ways, recovering alcoholics don't usually have well-stocked drinks trolleys. It's not exactly helpful.

Belinda stopped blaming herself for being weak. She suddenly understood why she cheated, and was able to be kinder to herself. She still eats sugar, but is more aware of how addictive she finds it.

It's only natural that we use substances to make ourselves feel better, and to ease our way through life. We have been doing it since time began, whether with alcohol, tobacco, highly palatable food or drugs. It can be hard to stop. It's very much a personal decision how you decide to deal with this - whether to cut down quantity, completely ignore it, or start a lobby group to get governments to take action.

I no longer work for food companies because it didn't sit well with me. That was my decision.

ACTION

What is your relationship with certain foods? Do you use them to medicate yourself?

How does this make you feel about manufactured food? Does it change your opinion of them?

Could you choose to moderate your intake?

You saw it so you want it

Pavlov is well known for his experiments regarding dogs. When he fed them, he rang a little bell. Eventually, he only needed to ring the bell and the dogs salivated, even when there was no food.

I know we'd like to think that we're superior to dogs. But there are lots of things in our lives that act like this trigger. Events that induce salivation due to habit. It might be turning on the television, if you usually eat in front of it. Or driving past a garage if you buy snacks when you fill up. Or walking past a certain bakery if you often buy cakes there.

You weren't thinking of eating a cinnamon roll, were you, until you walked past the bakery and that delicious sweet, spicy smell engulfed you? All at once, your tongue tingles with the anticipation of the sugary coating, the warm, yeasty bread beneath. You find yourself in the shop. A moment earlier you weren't even hungry.

Or maybe you're watching television and there is Nigella, dipping her finger into an oozing mass of chocolatey sauce. All at once, the idea of chocolate, or Nutella or a hot pudding fills your mind. The next thing you know, you're on the hunt for it.

What in your life, acts like that bell, and has you salivating for food whether you're hungry or not? Can you retrain the dog?

I love the introduction to the scientific paper called Eating with our Eyes: "One of the brain's key roles is to facilitate foraging and feeding. It is presumably no coincidence, then, that the mouth is situated close to the brain in most animal species."

The mouth is close to the brain, indeed! This same paper talks of 'food porn'. We are currently obsessed with images of food. Instagram feeds are crammed with photographs of meals and snacks. Cookery channels dominate television with depictions of luscious ingredients whisked into appetising meals. Food has become more forbidden than sex. We are ogling pictures of it in the same way that men used to sneak glances at 1970's centrefolds.

In America, digital media influences more than 70 percent of the food eaten by households. Research show that "external food cues, such as the sight of appetizing food can evoke a desire to eat, even in the absence of hunger." Again - no kidding... these scientists seem to spend years researching things that you and I knew to be true from a relatively young age.

What's really interesting is that physical things happen, just from seeing a picture. We salivate (we all know that). But more worryingly, we produce insulin. Our bodies shoot out the hormone required to deal with the sugar even when we haven't eaten it. And of course, when our insulin goes up, we crave sugar even more to balance it out. Even our heart rate goes up in anticipation of the food.

This is where we need to track back to chapter two on hunger. Food manufacturers know that seductive images of delicious food will draw us in, hungry or not. And our brains, as we have seen from the section on unconscious behaviours, will take the trigger and act on it, without even consulting our conscious selves.

A German study asked 50 volunteers to wear a blindfold while they ate ice cream and compared their reactions with those who saw what they ate. The blindfolded group rated the ice cream as less palatable and pleasant than those who could see what they were eating. They also ate slightly less, but estimated that they had consumed a lot more.

Another small study found a similar phenomenon when participants had a lunchtime meal. Those who were blindfolded ate 22 percent less food than the control group, but reported feeling just as full.

It could be that there is some truth to that old expression that: "Your eyes are bigger than your stomach." In other words, if food looks appealing, you could be driven to take more of it, and maybe also eat more of it. It does seem a tad extreme, however, to turn up to a restaurant with a blindfold and insist on eating that way, regardless of wine glasses flying left and right and food ending up on your lap.

Nonetheless, there's something here worth pondering. We use all our senses when we eat, and when we remove one of them, we enjoy it less and therefore tend to consume less of it.

If we can be mindful, and stop for a moment and think about whether we are hungry, then we can ask ourselves if we really want to eat. Consider the chapter on satisfaction and fullness. If we aren't hungry when we start eating, how do we know when to stop?

If you find yourself drawn to a food because you have just seen it or a picture of it, someone else is eating it or you walked past a shop selling it... stop and ask yourself: Do I really want it now? I can have it now, or tomorrow? If I promise myself ten servings of it tomorrow, do I want it now?

This is another trick that Belinda used. She would feel devastated at the thought of never eating sugar again. And this sense of deprivation would drive her to eat it today 'because I can't have it tomorrow'.

So Belinda turned this on its head. She told herself: "Tomorrow I will eat ten kilograms of chocolate." The thought of this was slightly nauseating, and put her off eating any today. But she told herself that she genuinely could eat ten kilograms tomorrow. When tomorrow came, she didn't want ten kilograms, so she promised it to herself the next day. In this way, she found that she only really wanted chocolate now and then, and when she did, she allowed herself to have it.

If we know that cues in our environment can trigger our desire to eat something, its worth reviewing what surrounds us. If a mere picture of food is enough to make us want to eat it, when we might not otherwise have thought of it, then keeping our homes relatively free of that makes it easier not to 'cheat'. You might have a cupboard at eye level and when you open it, the first thing you see is chocolate. Or perhaps the biscuits are stored next to the tea, so whenever you make a cup of tea you see the biscuits, which will create a desire to eat one.

Leave a chocolate cake on the counter? Of course you'll want to eat it. If it's in a plastic tub in a cupboard, it will be less tempting.

ACTION

Where you can, control your environment so that you aren't surrounded by tempting images.

If you keep foods that you find hard to resist at home, store them somewhere that you don't normally use. Don't put them in a high traffic area - that's a recipe for disaster.

Think of Pavlov and his dogs. What in your life, acts like that bell, and has you salivating for food whether you're hungry or not? Can you retrain the dog?

Because I ate while doing something else

Michael is a delightful restaurant owner – he is the epitome of what you might imagine – jolly, jovial, larger than life. And you might be forgiven for assuming that the larger than life part is due to the abundance of food in his restaurants.... Think again. Because every night, on his way home from the restaurant, he buys a 1kg bar of Dairy Milk, and consumes the lot.

Perhaps you've done it? You've just filled up with petrol, and somehow a bar of chocolate is in your lap, bought in a rush, an impulse at the checkout. You fumble at it, fingers slipping on the wrapper as you try to keep your hands on the steering wheel, heart pounding. You glance at the other drivers. They aren't looking at you, their focus is on the road. Unlike yours. Your focus is on the wrapper that isn't tearing.

You put both hands in your lap and rip, and the paper tears. Saliva rushes into your mouth like a dam breaking. The chocolate is already melting with the heat of your lap and the urgency of your desire. You break a piece off, the brown staining your fingertips as you cram it into your mouth. The traffic ahead stops sharply and you slam your foot down, pulse racing as you swallow down the sticky sweetness.

A long drive, you might think? Maybe a two hour commute where he's hungry and needs sustenance? That's not the case – his drive is approximately ten minutes. Maybe fifteen if the traffic is bad (which, by the time he leaves the restaurant, it never is). And in that time, during that brief drive, he ate (although I'm not sure this is the best word – perhaps inhaled?) a kilogram of chocolate.

Did he really taste it? Did he enjoy it? Did he focus on it? Or did he shove it down as fast as he could so that no-one would know?

When Michael came to see me, he told me this, with a bit of a giggle: laughter to cover his shame. He knew what the problem was, he just couldn't stop it.

Eating in the car is a common way to 'cheat'. This is a place where no one can see. Aside from other drivers, and they don't count.

I can recall eating a large muffin in the car. While stopped at traffic lights, I realised that a lorry driver was leering down at me. I thought for a brief moment that my skirt had ridden up until I looked down. My top was strewn with crumbs and pieces of cake. I still remember the hot burning flush of shame that fell over me, my face so warm that it could have melted the windscreen.

Nobody who eats in cars, has ever told me that they enjoyed the food that they ate. Some could hardly recall what they had eaten; others stuffed it down so fast that they didn't even taste it. One said that every mouthful tasted of shame.

We can eat while watching television or at the movies, or while working - to ease away the afternoon. When we looked at how people 'cheat' on their eating resolutions, doing so in a distracted manner is one of the most common ways. It's as though if we aren't concentrating on it, it doesn't count.

So how much can you eat while distracted? How much food can you put away 'without noticing' - the answer is: A lot.

Scientists have turned this on its head. They investigated how much we might eat if we had already pictured ourselves eating a load of that food. You might suspect this would increase cravings yet in reality, the opposite seems to occur.

The participants imagined performing 33 repetitive motions: Half of them imagined eating 30 M&Ms and inserting three quarters into the slot of a laundry machine. The other half envisioned eating three M&Ms and inserting 30 quarters. Then everyone was allowed to eat their fill from a bowl of M&Ms. Those who'd envisioned eating more candy ate about three M&Ms on average (or about 2.2 grams), whereas the others ate about five M&Ms (or about 4.2 grams).

Just as an aside, I find this hard to believe that anyone ate just three M&Ms, let alone undergraduate students. Most people find it hard to stop at five. But the starving students of the world? If they'd asked me to participate when I was at University, I suspect I would eaten the entire bowl.

Anyway... the research didn't stop there. They extended their findings to cheese. As in the M&M experiment, those who imagined eating 30 cheese cubes consumed less of the real thing. Then they mixed it up, so that the participants imagined M&Ms and got offered cheese, at which point it didn't matter whether they'd imagined eating three M&Ms or thirty - they all ate the same amount of cheese. Thus, the habituation effect seems to be specific to the type of food imagined. If you picture eating lots of chocolate, it won't save you from the cheese platter, and vice versa.

On follow-up questionnaires, they found that the mental imagery doesn't diminish how much the participants liked a particular food, but in a final experiment, in which they played a computer game to earn cheese cubes, it seemed that it might reduce the effort people will expend to get food.

How about turning using this to help us lose weight?

What if you knew that tomorrow you had to eat two kilograms of chocolate and three tubs of ice cream all in one sitting. Imagine it. Really think what that would be like. Forcing down more chocolate after you had already eaten a kilogram.

If that was on the menu for tomorrow, would you want to eat chocolate today? If you knew you could eat all that you wanted both tomorrow and every day thereafter, would it be so critical to eat that much of it today? Later, we'll look at an experiment where they did just that.

One possible strategy might be to spend a few minutes before each meal imagining eating exactly the foods we're about to consume. This type of mental exercise might also help counter sudden cravings between meal times. Given that many diets urge people to suppress thoughts of the foods they crave and that usually doesn't work, how about imagining eating all those forbidden foods.

ACTION

Rather than reaching for the food you're not allowing yourself, imagine eating it. Try to focus on the sensation, the taste, the texture. Summon up the experience of putting it into your mouth, of chewing it, swallowing. Keep going, eating mouthful after mouthful.

As you continue, do you find you want it more or less?

Summary

Our brains have automated programs they can switch on with a single taste, or even a single thought about foods we often overeat. This is a useful feature that normally allows us to drive to work while thinking about other things. it's not so useful when it comes to managing our eating.

Try to recognise which thoughts or foods might set off a cavalcade of actions over which you have little control, or consciousness. As we are also triggered by what we see around us, think about what foods you have on display and where you keep them. Make it easier for yourself by ensuring you don't come face to face with a large bar of chocolate every time you want a glass of water.

Accept that food manufacturers are using every trick in the book to create addiction to their foods. Every part of our brains and bodies are seduced by the heady combination of sugar salt and fat. Decide how much you want to buy into this. You don't have to give these foods up, but knowing the effects they have on us, you may want to consider them more as drugs than as nutritious meals.

Weight loss is slow, and can't compete with the immediate and overwhelming reward of food, especially the high sugar, high fat foods. Stay in touch with your hunger and what you really want. When it is time to eat, really focus on your food and ensure that you feel satisfied.

Give yourself permission to enjoy what you eat.

CHAPTER FIVE
OUR BELIEF SYSTEMS

We are fed an awful lot of misinformation when it comes to healthy eating, dieting, and our bodies. Some of it is with the best of intentions. A new guideline is announced and then science makes another discovery and the advice we had been following is proved wrong.

But an awful lot of it is designed to sell more diet plans and to make us less and less reliant on ourselves and our bodies, and more reliant on external rules.

All of this history of dieting and failing, combined with the many conflicting messages out there, can mean that we feel quite hopeless and helpless when it come to eating healthily or losing weight.

Our belief systems can support us or they can undermine us. This is about throwing away the ones that aren't working, and moving towards a more positive frame of mind.

I failed last time and broke the diet

"I was trying to lose weight, and we had this long meeting, and someone brought in a box of doughnuts. These doughnuts, they just sat on the table and looked at me, the way a doughnut can stare you down, daring me to look away, locking my eyes in a battle to the death, challenging me. Well, I never met a doughnut I didn't like, and after they sat on the table for a while, taunting me, I caved in. I can

Malcolm, 52

The moment that you pop something into your mouth that isn't on the detox or healthy eating plan, your brain explodes. Not literally. It explodes into action with thoughts of guilt and failure. "Why did I eat that?" "I may as well give up now." "I've broken the diet."

These thoughts can pull you into a tunnel of despair. "I'll never lose weight." "I deserve to be fat." "Everyone else can do it except me." And the tunnel can get darker and darker until it colours everything in your world. "My life is hopeless." "No one will ever date me." "Who could love a failure like me?" The belief that we can't succeed in losing weight, or eating healthily is like a cloud that can make the rest of our lives look grey. Our job prospects appear less rosy, our love lives suffer. All because we've had a mouthful of something that we believe we shouldn't.

It's amazing how one bite can 'break' a diet. It's pretty fragile if a single mouthful leads to total collapse. Imagine you bought a sofa, and if you crossed your legs, the sofa crumbled beneath you. If that happened, you'd want your money back. If a new dress split down all the seams when you took a deep breath - you'd be furious. (or embarrassed. I once walked across the city, thinking how cool and breezy it was, before I realised that my skirt had split completely up the back and everyone could see my underwear.)

Diets, detox plans, healthy eating plans - call them what you like. They can't be very robust if a mouthful leads to their undoing. This is one of the issues with them - they are black and white. You are on them or off them. Virtuous or vile. Clean eating and included, or unclean and outcast, a leper.

Then there's that point just before the diet starts. I like to call it 'The Last Supper'. Or stuffing your face because you can't have it tomorrow

Greta tells me of how she would sit on the sofa reading the book about the detox that starts tomorrow. There is a flutter of excitement in her tummy. This is it! At long last she is going to be healthy and thin. She reads the pages again - the program sounds do-able. She nods to herself. This time it will be different. This time, she will stick to the program. Her energy will soar, her skin will be clear, her hair thick and lustrous. It's the right thing to do for her body, for her health.

Well, she tells herself, if she is dieting tomorrow, she may as well have the chocolate today, because she won't be having it for three weeks. A bar of chocolate later, her mouth feels too sweet. She needs something salty to balance it out. There's no point in denying herself some chips. She won't be eating them again for a while, dammit. She crams the crisps into her mouth.

Sometimes, the sense of approaching deprivation can be so great that the feeding frenzy lasts days before the next detox or eating plan. The detox feels like a lifeboat in a choppy sea of endless eating that threatens to drown us. Unless we cling on to the rigid restrictions of the diet, there will be no end to the hunger, no end to the weight that piles onto our bodies.

The problem with this argument, is that it is the very thought and act of restriction, deprivation and hunger, that drives this uncontrolled eating. Science has proved this time and again. The experiment mentioned right at the beginning of the book - where perfectly healthy men were driven to over-eating, bingeing, food obsessions and poring over recipe books? It only took a restrictive diet to do that, and the ramifications lasted for many months after the experiment ended. Let's not repeat that experiment on ourselves for the rest of our lives. We've proven it enough times. Without the dieting, there wouldn't be the panicked over-eating.

There is a saying that we are what we think and it can be true that how we think about things shapes both us and what happens to us. If we believe something will happen to us - we will 'manifest' it. This is because our attitudes and beliefs shape how we each interact with the world. They provide a lens through which we view the world and interpret what is happening to us. They provide a frame also that assists us with making decisions and forming judgments.

Our attitude to and beliefs about food, weight and eating are major factors in our health and wellbeing. They affect if and how we lose weight, as well as when and how we encounter difficulties and overcome them. They affect how we feel about our bodies, how we respond to cues to eat and external pressures. They may even change our views on exercise and which foods we might like to eat.

We are fed lots of new beliefs with all of the diets that come out. These beliefs might include:

"Carbohydrates will make you fat"

"Thighs should be thin"

"Fat will make you fat"

"Weight loss is easy"

"Weight loss is hard"

"Eating late at night will make you fat."

"Anyone can stick to a diet"

"I can't lose weight, I'm destined not to be slim."

"If you can't stick to a diet, it's because you don't have willpower"

All of these and many more attitudes and beliefs shape our world and affect our success at managing a healthy body weight. Fundamentally, there is only one thing that makes us fat – eating too much. Equally, there is only one thing that keeps us slim – eating the amount that your body needs. These attitudes and beliefs just cloud the issue and make it harder to eat when we are hungry and harder to stop when we are full. There may be a feeling of deprivation if you leave something on your plate, even if you are full. Or anxiety if you don't finish off the chocolate, because you don't know when you next might have some.

It might be really difficult to stop labelling food as 'good' or 'bad'. After all, we have had years of being told that chocolate is bad. Chips are bad. Cucumber is good. Which isn't much help if you don't like cucumber. (I don't really, unless it's chopped small in something else. For that matter, I don't much like celery either).

The thing to remember is that a belief is only a belief. It isn't a fact. If you have a mouthful of ice cream, you may believe that you have broken your diet, but it doesn't mean that you can't lose weight. That's an illogical conclusion - a catastrophic extension of a small act. If I eat a mouthful of ice cream, then I'll never lose weight. Obviously, if you eat a lot of mouthfuls of ice cream, it's going to make it harder, but you can still lose weight. Recently, a personal trainer committed to eating just ice cream for ten days. He didn't lose weight, but he certainly lost his taste for ice cream, and he wasn't fatter at the end of it all. In fact, there are various examples of people (it does seem to be largely men) who have lost weight on an ice cream only diet.

You may have failed last time. Perhaps it was because you chose the difficult route, the way that didn't really suit you. It was the diet's fault.

Changing beliefs is quite hard - they are often founded early in life, and we tend to interpret things that happen to us in a way that reinforces the beliefs rather than challenges them. But to get around them, sometimes you don't have to change them. Sometimes you can just dismiss them as a belief and not a fact.

If you believe that you can't lose weight because you failed last time, that is a belief, not a fact. You could choose to prove the belief wrong.

If you believe that you can't stop at one doughnut, then there are several options open to you. Either try and put yourself out of the way of temptation, or investigate why you can't stop. Is it because of some of the physiological reasons that we've explored - that a priming has occurred in your body, and you are now driven by cravings to continue eating? Even if that is the case, if your life depended on it, you could stop.

It's time to challenge some of the beliefs that we have about ourselves and food especially the negative ones. Diets and eating plans feed off these, making us feel ever more powerless, and ever more in thrall to another set of rules. It's time to stand up to beliefs that aren't helping us, to start trusting ourselves and ignoring all those outside voice that think they might know better.

They don't.

ACTION

A bite doesn't break anything. A bite is a bite. You can do anything you choose when it comes to eating and your health.

Make a list of your beliefs about food, eating and your body. Decide which ones are helpful and what you might be prepared to let go.

Experiment with promising things for tomorrow versus allowing them today.

If you are unsure whether or not you want chocolate/crisps/a certain food today, trying promising yourself that you will eat it tomorrow, and see how you feel.

Crazy Diets: Jackie Onassis

Jackie Onassis would eat one baked potato a day stuffed with beluga caviar and soured cream.

She watched the scales "with the rigour of a diamond merchant counting his carats", according to her social secretary Tish Baldrige. If she went a couple of pounds over her usual weight, she would fast for a day, then confine herself to a diet of fruit until she was back to normal.

The bites that 'don't count'

Perhaps you turned down a slice of cake, but now you find yourself at the plate, knife in hand, just making sure that the edge is even. You cut a sliver and shove it into your mouth. The cake tastes delicious. You return to the platter and ease off another morsel. Now the edge is a mess. You take the knife again and cut to smooth the ends. A short while later, the cake is considerably smaller...

It's very easy to say that one mouthful won't make a difference. The question is then, which mouthful makes us fat? Is it the first? Or the hundredth?

Maybe your friends are saying, come on, you've done really well! One dessert won't kill you! They are right, it won't, but it's very easy for that one dessert to become many.

There are many times we can tell ourselves 'This doesn't count'. I didn't order a dessert - I ate if from my husband's plate, so that doesn't count. Or I was just clearing dishes, and it was a shame to let the rest go to waste. So I scoffed it rather than put it in the garbage.

It's much easier to let ourselves off the hook than stick to a diet because diets require us to make a huge effort. They ask for such a large change. Everything we know, everything we do is thrown out of the window. Your normal eating habits are utterly disrupted to make way for a new miracle fix that promises amazing results.

This is mainly because most of us believe that losing weight is so hard, so painful and so mysterious, that only the truly radical solutions will work.

But what if that wasn't the case at all? What if one tiny change was all that was needed?

I used to think that one tiny change would never result in the loss of the fifteen kilos that I wanted to shed. To lose that kind of weight, a change had to be dramatic, drastic, and most of all, tortuous.

Medical research is showing that is not the case at all. They examined the world's fattest man, and to reach his astronomical weight, all you have to do is eat 300 calories more than you need, every day, for about twenty years. He was so large that they had to take him to hospital on a forklift truck. So basically, all you need to do, to become enormously fat, is to eat one Mars Bar too many, every day. Gosh, I thought. That's so easy to do! I could easily eat a small bar of chocolate more than I need every day. And some days, I could eat several.

Luckily, the reverse is also true.

If you reduce you calories a little bit every day, even if only by 50, you will lose weight. That's just one biscuit. If you eat one biscuit less, every day, over the course of a year, you'll lose weight. About five pounds or two kilograms, to be exact.

None of us think of it like that. The reason is that when we're eating, we only really think of today:

"I'll just have dessert today as it's my birthday"

"I'll have cake as it's Colleen's birthday at work"

"I'll have another glass of wine as I had a hard day today"

And what many of us don't recognise is that every day, we have an excuse or a reason to eat more than we need. With 365 days in a year, those extra 100 calories a day, add up to 36,500 calories in a year. That's more than ten pounds of extra weight.

Conversely, if you cut out just 100 calories of your normal diet, you will create a deficit of ten pounds or five kilos a year. A year, I hear you cry. You can't possibly wait a whole year to lose five kilos. In which case, it might be time to take a different approach. If you've lost and regained the same ten pounds or twenty kilos as many times as most of us, how about taking a year to lose it and never getting it back?

Eat your usual diet and food, and just cut out two biscuits, or one piece of toast. No huge changes. No fancy shakes, meal plans and weighing. Just one small change.

If you can't face a massive effort, can you manage that?

Other things that 'don't count' are foods labelled as 'healthy', 'low fat' or 'sugar free'. We hope this means that it won't impact our waistlines.

Part of the problem with the 'fat free' messages of the 1990s, is that we all thought that if there wasn't any fat, we could eat an unlimited amount. It's fairly safe to say that several million people have proved otherwise. You can definitely get fat on 'fat free', largely because the fat has been replaced by sugar.

Likewise 'sugar free' or 'paleo' - these diets recommend very high calorie foods, with the suggestion that because they don't contain sugar, you won't get fat. The messages are that as long as you stick to the guidelines, then the quantity doesn't matter. Sadly, overeating high-fat low-sugar foods will still lead to weight gain, just the same as overeating fat-free high-sugar foods,.

A top Sydney nutritionist, Catherine Saxelby, compared the two bounty bars. The sugar-free 'healthy' ones, and the ones you buy in the shops. Her analysis shows that the two have about the same number of calories. The 'healthy' ones have twice the amount of saturated fat. She says: "We were pleasantly surprised with the look of the 'Healthy Bounty Bar', particularly the dark chocolate colour and the moist centre. However, this initial promise of delight was let down once we bit into it. Most kindly described as 'neutral' in flavour, there was no standout coconut or chocolate flavour. It was rich, due to the large amount of coconut oil used (a whole jar for the recipe!), but strangely, not satisfying.' She goes on to clarify "It's still not sugar-free, just sucrose-free which is not the same."

It's all too easy to 'cheat', telling ourselves that it's 'healthy' to eat bliss balls, or raw oat bars, or paleo cakes. These things may (or may not, as we've just seen) be healthier than the alternatives. But our bodies don't see things in this light. Our bodies take calories and either burn them or store them as fat. It doesn't matter whether the surplus calories come from a cereal bar Nestle produced in a factory or one you made in your kitchen, or one that an expensive Paleo cafe rustled up. Our bodies don't care where it was made or what's in it, in terms of calories, if we eat too much, we'll put on weight. The 'healthy' label doesn't mean it doesn't count.

Nutritionally, it is, of course, better for our bodies to have something with more vitamins, minerals and fibre included.

Calling a food healthy, or telling ourselves that 'this doesn't count' are ways that we give ourselves permission to eat more than we know is healthy for us. This doesn't matter if we do it occasionally. It's just that these days, we are surrounded by so many opportunities to eat, that it can be very hard to decide what counts and what doesn't and very easy to do something that 'doesn't count' every day.

The best way is to keep in touch with our natural sense of hunger, and to think about what we really want to eat. Perhaps, when it's Colleen's birthday and there is a large cake, you aren't that hungry. Or you're getting hungry, but it isn't really cake that you want to eat. Give yourself permission to have cake when you want it, so that you don't need to have it every time you're offered it, just in case there isn't a 'next time'.

I'm so confused about which rules to follow

"Aren't you going to have rules for people to follow?" asked Anita when we were discussing my progress with this book. "People love rules."

"I know," I sighed, "But rules are what get most people into trouble And most of the rules put of there in diet books are total bollocks, and I can't bear for people to go to all this trouble following guidelines that aren't helping them at all. Besides, most people, once they have rules, then bend or break them."

"I like rules," said Anita firmly, "And I stick to them. I have two crackers if I have a workout and only one if I don't."

"Well, you're weird," I answered. (She is an accountant)

"I still think you should have rules," she said.

So here they are - many of the rules I could find:

Snacking is unhealthy

Eating small meals keeps your metabolism high

Veganism is good for you - don't eat meat

Paleo is good for you - eat meat!

Drink two litres of water a day

Don't drink while you eat

Saturated fat is bad

Eat lots of fibre

Don't eat carbohydrates after 8pm

Eat a large breakfast

Fast until noon

Only eat fruit before lunchtime

Skipping a meal will wreck your blood sugar

Fasting regularly will help your blood sugar

Sugar is bad

Eat ten serves of fruit and vegetables a day. or was that five? or seven?

Dairy will kill you

Nuts are fattening

Nuts are good for you

Breakfast is the most important meal of the day.

Don't eat after 8pm.

Avoid carbs and eat meat.

Avoid meat and go vegan.

Don't eat gluten.

Eat lots of small meals a day.

Eat three meals a day and two snacks

Don't snack.

Fast all day and eat one meal in the evening.

How are we supposed to know what to do? Each of these rules has either so-called scientific backing, or evidence of people who have lost weight following it, until we are completely befuddled. A new plan comes out each week telling us that we have it all wrong and if only we do it a different way, then we'll lose weight.

The rules keep changing for several reasons. The main one is that nutrition and science behind what we should eat is very complex and very difficult to research. It is almost impossible to tell, even in a carefully controlled experiment, whether one person lost weight because they ate low fat, or because they exercised more. You can't account for genetic differences, for what people do outside the laboratory environment that they don't tell you about, for how much exercise they do. Then there are other factors like pollution, smoking, alcohol, the interaction with drugs that each person might be taking, and it's almost absurd to believe we can point the finger at a single thing like fat or sugar.

We are such complex beings, a mixture of body, mind and spirit, of behaviours and gut bacteria, of brains and anatomy, or varying systems in that anatomy, that finding out the reason for any particular change, especially weight loss or gain, is very hard. So scientists make up a hypothesis, do their best to test it, and then publish the results. Other scientists have different ideas, test those, and then publish conflicting results. One of the things I've tried to do here, is to amalgamate all the research from all the different fields.

There is one rule that we know works for weight loss: eat less. And most of these other rules are just ways of getting you to do just that. The only challenge is that sometimes eating less feels very difficult.

Often, that's because as soon as you try to adhere to other people's rules, rules that don't suit you at all, then you're likely to fail. And then you're back on the diet - failure - hate yourself loop.

So why not question the rules? All of them.

I rarely feel hungry first thing, so I often don't eat breakfast. So far, it has neither killed me, nor led to me putting on weight. On the contrary, I wait until I am hungry, and then eat, which puts me in tune with my body.

I got so confused as to whether I should ditch carbs and just eat meat (Atkins diet) or ditch the meat and go vegan, or whether it was dairy that was the problem or perhaps gluten, that I gave up. I gave up on all the external voices and listened to my own body.

My grandmother ate meat and dairy and gluten and sugar, and she was slim her entire life. This is true of most of our ancestors. So I threw out all the rules except these:

- Wait until you are hungry to eat
- Eat what you really want to eat, with your body, mind and spirit
- Focus on your food while you eat
- Stop when you have had enough

How about throwing out the rules along with your beliefs, and starting from scratch? That might sound scary. Perhaps you can just question one rule at a time, and see how that goes.

These rules aren't sacred. They aren't fixed in stone. Scientists question and retest them every day, and find new answers. It's up to us to do the same for ourselves.

Anita said later: "I've just realised that those are my rules. If someone else told me to do that, I'd rebel. But over time, I've discovered that this suits me. I am happy to stick to them, because I made them up." Exactly! It turns out, we are both saying the same thing. We each need to work out what suits us, not what works for others.

ACTION
Which rules to you need to break? Write them down and explore how you feel without them. Is it liberating? Or terrifying?

Which rules might help you?

Crazy Diets: Hunter S Thompson's breakfast

Journalist and author Hunter S Thompson describes his breakfast as "a personal ritual that can only be properly observed alone, and in a spirit of genuine excess.

"The food factor should always be massive: four Bloody Marys, two grapefruits, a pot of coffee, Rangoon crepes, a half-pound of either sausage, bacon or corned beef hash with diced chillies, a Spanish omelette or eggs Benedict, a quart of milk, a chopped lemon for random seasoning, and something like a slice of key lime pie, two margaritas, and six lines of the best cocaine for dessert ...

"All of which," he concluded, "should be dealt with outside, in the warmth of a hot sun, and preferably stone naked."

Why diets are still attractive, and your favourite foods are a bit scary

You fancy just one last time, don't you? One more diet or detox or healthy eating plan. You definitely won't cheat this time. And THEN, after that, you'll change the way you eat permanently.

When I was in thrall to food, I wrote in my journal:

I can't stop eating... three weeks now. What stops me from giving up the diets and eating normally is:
• Guilt from overeating in the last three weeks
• Terror at the weight I must have put on
• A feeling of helplessness and hopelessness that I'll ever lose it
• A consequent hatred of my body
• Disgust and despair at myself
Overeating acts both to blot out those feelings and to punish myself. If I felt attractive and glamorous and interesting, I wouldn't feel like bingeing. Instead I feel as though I don't deserve any better.

The terror of the weight, and the terror that my life might be one long endless binge without the constraints of an eating plan, kept me locked into diets, locked into their promise and hope, locked into their rigidity in a world where I didn't trust myself. Ironically, these diets and detox programs were the very thing preventing me from being a healthy weight. They were what had destroyed my self belief, and their rules had estranged me from my own body.

The lure, the promise that they make is almost irresistible. There are endless before and after photos, lists of science or pseudo-science that back up the claims. And each of us believes, or hopes that if only we could lose those kilograms/pounds, then everything would be alright.

Wouldn't it?

Diets and detoxes are fabulous because they provide us with rules and restrictions. That makes them easy to follow and easy to believe in. We all want hard and fast rules, so that we don't have to decide for ourselves how much we should eat and whether or not we're really hungry. We also want guaranteed results, and the often photoshopped before and after pictures promise those.

But these are long term, sustainable behaviours. It's not what we want to eat and it usually requires us to give up what we love.

Which brings us to the question: what do you really love to eat? Do you actually know? Has it all become confused with what you should and should not be eating?

I'm not sure about you, but I don't want to be lying on my deathbed wishing that I had eaten more ice cream on holiday, or thinking of years wasted struggling with some weird lemon and paprika drink (Beyonce) when I could have had a lovely chicken and mayonnaise sandwich.

Life is too short to eat celery.

Whatever it is that you love, make sure that you eat it! But here is the challenging part: with all the messages around food, do you know what you really love? Do you really love doughnuts, or cake? Or is it just that they are forbidden, so you sneak them because you believe you aren't allowed them? Have you ever really stopped and tasted them? And then observed how your body feels afterwards?

It's worth finding out what you really enjoy eating. Then make sure you eat as much of it as you feel like.

The important word here is 'enjoy'. This means sitting down, looking at and anticipating the food in front of you. Maybe even drooling a little. Smelling it, feeling the saliva build in your mouth. Tasting just a tiny bit and letting the delightful sensation spread across your body. Experience the anticipation that there is more to come. It means eating slowly, relishing every mouthful. And at some point, feeling as though that will do very nicely, thank you, and pushing back your chair and stopping.

Notice how your body responds. How is your energy afterwards? A few hours later? Has your mood changed and if so how? (Sugar has been shown to be linked to depression - which is certainly depressing considering how many of us eat it to cheer ourselves up.)

Enjoy does not mean cramming 'forbidden' foods down as quickly as possible before someone sees. Or quickly fingering the remnants from someone else's plate into your mouth, because you didn't 'deserve' a portion of your own. Enjoying implies permission: permission to take pleasure in eating, permission to decide exactly what you'd like to eat, and permission to take your time and leisure in savouring every taste.

Really looking at which foods you enjoy can be quite enlightening. For example, there may be so called diet foods, that you 'had to eat', such a salads, or chicken, that you discover that you really enjoy eating, when you give yourself permission to eat whatever you choose. There may be other foods that you thought you enjoyed, that when you sit down and really taste them, you find to be sickly sweet. Or perhaps they make you feel bloated afterwards and this spoils the pleasure.

Finding out what you enjoy is a slow and delightful process. Every meal is another opportunity to fully taste what is in front of you and see whether you like it, see how it sits in your body, how you feel after the meal. And if you don't like it, I recommend that you don't eat it. Why on earth would you want to eat anything that you don't like? Why waste the calories? If you aren't enjoying it, stop. There will be another meal (I promise). There are better alternatives.

When I really paid attention, I found that raspberries and cream were more delightful to me than chocolate. Chocolate was sometimes too sweet and too cloying in the mouth. Whereas the tangy sweetness of the raspberries with the smoothness of the cream - divine! I still enjoy chocolate, but not as often as I thought I might.

As you eat slowly and with appreciation, your body will start asking for certain foods. I gave up red meat for a long time, and after I had reintroduced it into my diet a couple of times, I found my body asking for it, not often, but perhaps twice a year. I would get a craving for a really rich, hearty, meaty stew. Maybe my body needed iron, or protein, or something else. But once I had eaten and savoured the stew, that would be it for another few months.

Try and increase your concentration on your meal or food as you eat it. Is the taste of it really tickling your tongue? Or when you really focus on it, is it not quite what you thought it would be? How is the texture for you – too soft? Crisp and crunchy? Do you enjoy the way it is making you feel? Over time, focus on what foods delight you, and then make sure you give yourself the time and the opportunity to delight in them.

Conversely, if you are not enjoying a specific food, why eat it? Well, you might be polite if someone has cooked it for you. But even then, why eat it? Gently pushing it to one side should not break friendships.

Greta, who we met earlier, used to cycle between eating clean and cheat days but would massively overeat on the cheat days, until she felt she couldn't trust herself around her favourite foods. For the past year, she has been focused on her hunger and her eating enjoyment.

She's been practising "Eating Just Enough" with both foods she has regarded as 'clean' and those she regarded as 'treats'. She can't let go of the labels just yet, but is able to experiment with leaving room for treats in case she wants to have one. She's noticed that, since she can have treats whenever she wants she no longer feels like she "loses control" when she's around treats. She's practised starting and stopping having treats, and now trusts herself to do so. She really likes how she feels now. She likes that she can listen to her body and stop when she's full. She also knows that some foods are harder to stop eating, so she makes sure she doesn't buy too many of those, or she only has them with friends.

Before, eating her 'danger foods' would often often completely get away from her if she was feeling sad, bored, or tired. Now, she has them when she wants them, and she really enjoys them. Interestingly, this has spilled out into the rest of her life, and she takes better care of herself in general.

There is something indulgent about eating our favourite foods every day, and most of us could do with a little more indulgence in our lives. Many of us, when we explore what we like to eat, find that our favourite foods range from the healthy to the less good for us, and that's absolutely fine. It's fine to like both mangoes and chocolate, or doughnuts and prawns. Once again, these things are personal, and are influenced by our childhoods, our cultures, our experiences throughout life.

The important thing is to increase our enjoyment of food. It shouldn't be a punishment. Because as soon as we feel punished, we'll cheat.

ACTION

Give yourself permission to enjoy food and take time to savour it.

Start looking at the aspects of food you enjoy, or things that you feel like: salty or sweet, crunchy or chewy or soft? Warm or cool?

See then how your body feels afterwards. Does it feel pleasantly full? Do you feel energized? Or are you now lethargic? Does your stomach feel bloated or still comfortable? Do you want to feel this way again? By really examining how you ARE after eating, you will better be able to gauge what the next meal will do for you, and how you may want to adjust that in future.

Make a list of your favourite foods and ensure you eat them all regularly. Keep adding to it over the days and weeks so that you have a long list of everything that you really enjoy eating. Notice which flavours or textures re-occur in your list. See whether you prefer different foods at different times of the day or the year.

Promise yourself to try not to continue eating something that you are not enjoying.

Eat something you love at every meal.

Because I'll never have my dream body

You tell yourself that you could have your dream body, that you SHOULD have your dream body if only you worked hard enough (if only you could be bothered). Slim, lithe, toned, just the right amount of muscle definition. Lightly tanned. No bulges or bumps. It's just a question of eating better and exercising more. It's just a question of self control, being a bit more disciplined.

Self control? I feel tired just thinking about it. Who has the energy for that? Discipline? Didn't we leave that behind at school?

Perhaps you feel it is lurking inside you, just temporarily covered by a layer of adipose tissue. All it needs is an archaeologist to come and uncover it - or a lover, or the right diet or eating plan. This is because we're sold the myth that if we don't have the perfect body then it must be our fault. Somehow we're too lazy, greedy, or just plain bad to have it.

We're told that anyone can be young slim and beautiful. Madonna is touted as an example of what can be achieved with diet and exercise (well, she used to be - things have turned slightly weird recently). Gwyneth Paltrow, the goddess of clean, offers the promise of beauty that comes with health and 'clean' eating and living. (No mention of her genetic inheritance, which is, lets face it, pretty spectacular.) Magazines are full of young, firm, tanned bodies. The television is spawning more and more programmes on weight loss, makeovers, and cosmetic surgery until we believe that we aren't 'right' unless our bodies are perfect.

Bodies were not made 'perfect' or to order. For a start, the notion of perfection has varied dramatically over the centuries - from the Rubenesque curves of a couple of centuries ago, to the pallor of the Victorians, to the tans of the 1970's. Beauty really has been in the eye of the beholder. The ideals of beauty may vary over time, but the message remains the same: woe betide those who don't conform to their century's or decade's image.

In the 1950s we were supposed to be curvaceous, and a scant ten years later, our curves were expected to vanish so that we could adopt the 'Twiggy' boyish figure. It's hard to tell, these days, whether we are supposed to have Kim Kardashian's bottom or abs of steel. Perhaps both?

Is this a way to treat ourselves? Bodies are fragile, fallible things. They bleed if cut. They fatten if overfed. They die if starved.

Bodies are the means through which we experience the world. They allow us to walk, talk, kiss, and make babies. Through them we see sunsets, smell flowers, and listen to rock bands or Beethoven. They were never designed for their appearance. They were designed for the amazing things that they can do and experience. Sometimes, we don't appreciate these things until we've lost them. We don't appreciate our health until the moment we get a cold, and then we are indignant at the struggle to breathe, as we cough and sneeze our way through the day. A few days earlier, we hadn't thought twice about breathing deeply and comfortably.

We all take the ability to walk for granted, until we twist an ankle or are brought down with back pain that reduces us to a limping stagger.

Perhaps it's time that we made friends with our bodies, that we sat down and thanked them for everything that they'd done for us - digesting our food, seeing the world, carrying the shopping, creating new cells that grow hair, repair skin, heal wounds.

We take more care of most things that we own than we do of our bodies. Our bodies are ignored until they break in some way and then we feel resentful. We expect them to carry on, swallowing whatever we put into them, functioning on minimal sleep, plagued by stress, sedentary when they'd rather be moving, and we expect them to do this without complaining.

Rather than wait for the body to break down, or start aching, it might make sense to look after it a little.

It can be important to notice how your body feels. Not what it looks like, but the messages it's sending to you. Is it hot or cold, are parts of it aching? Do you have a surge of energy some days? What do you ask of your body?

Are there ways you could take care of it better? Perhaps you need a little more sleep, or that nap I mentioned earlier. Maybe the kids could tidy their own rooms, or god forbid, live with them messy, so that you get a little time to yourself. Perhaps another hour surfing the internet might be better spent walking in the Spring sunshine, or going to bed earlier.

If we regard our bodies by how they look, and then dismiss them entirely because they will never live up to some unattainable ideal, where does that leave us? Certainly not in a place where we feel inclined to look after them.

For most of us, when we find a healthy weight that is sustainable, and we start working with the systems of our bodies, something miraculous happens. It stops feeling as though we are at war with our physical selves. We soften towards our bodies, feel less antagonistic or resentful towards them. We find ourselves more able to take care of them.

If we take better care of ourselves, it also means we can take better care of those who are important to us: our families and friends.

ACTION

Try to stop thinking of what your body looks like, and focus on what it feels like. How could you take better care of it, so that it functions better, and feels better?

Summary

Just because you have failed to stick to an eating plan in the past, doesn't mean that you can't do it. That's just a belief, not a fact. It was only true because you weren't working with your body's systems, you were working against them.

This time you get to choose the rules that you want to stick to. You can eat your favourite foods every day. You can eat at a time that you choose. You can stop when you have had enough.

As your blood sugar becomes stable, and the addictive programs in your brain run a little less, you'll find that the beliefs and rules you had around food change. The aren't set in stone. They are choices that you get to make every day.

CHAPTER SIX
LEARNED FOOD PREFERENCES
AND CULTURAL INFLUENCES

We learn what foods to like at a very young age. I have a Korean friend, and she loves Kimchi with everything. Kimchi is a pungent mix of cabbage, chilli, garlic, ginger - it's potent. To most westerners, it's a step too far, but if you've grown up in Korea, no meal is complete without it.

We also create associations with certain foods, either through our families or through experiences as we grow up.

All of these affect what we choose to eat and what we enjoy. Once again, an understanding of how these might be influencing our behaviour can allow us to consider our actions, and perhaps do something differently the next time.

Because I hate diet food

Many years ago, a scientist called Duncker devised a series of experiments. One of these was the white chocolate experiment. He flavoured a white chocolate powder with lemon so that it tasted sublime. Then he used valerian, a very bitter and unpleasant herbal root and mixed it with sugar. It was still pretty foul.

Children were read a story about a little field mouse, who hates one food - 'hemlock', a poison - and loves another - 'maple sugar'. When the mouse discovers maple sugar in a tree he realises he has 'never tasted such good stuff before'. The hemlock in the story is 'sour and disgusting'.

After the story, the children tasted some real 'hemlock' and 'maple sugar'. The hemlock or poison, was actually the white chocolate powder (not bitter at all). And the maple sugar was the nasty-tasting valerian. Yet when asked to choose the substance they preferred, two thirds of the children opted for the 'maple sugar'. The majority rejected the 'hemlock' even though many of them recognised that it tasted of chocolate. So let's just recap, the children actually preferred the foul one, just on the basis of a story.

Most of us believe that we are too old to be persuaded by a story about a mouse, however cute the mouse is. But the sad truth is that we are all still in thrall to memories: memories of being taken out for doughnuts or burgers with our Dad or of Mum cooking a birthday cake. Fast food and cakes get these associations with parties and fun, in a way that cucumber and lettuce never do.

Some people are forced to eat their vegetables, which means they never learn to love them - they are always the thing that you're 'supposed' to eat.

In my family, sweets were used as a reward. If you ate everything on your plate, you could have a piece of chocolate. If you were a 'good girl' then you could have a sweet. So what do I automatically turn to if I want to reward myself? The very thing that I have learned since birth is the best reward (because what your parents do is always the best...)... sugar.

It is possible to create new memories and associations with foods. Some people are forever repulsed by certain alcohols, if they drank them to excess and then threw up as a teenager. I know at least two middle-aged men who still can't drink whisky as it reminds them of vomiting into a gutter in their younger years.

I'm not suggested that you create associations around your favourite foods in such an extreme sense. But you might be able to develop new feelings for hitherto unexplored ingredients. A small passion for tomatoes, say, if you eat them at special times? Or a delight in mangos if they remind you of the summer?

If you look back, and see that you eat chocolate when you are lonely, or bored or somehow disappointed with life, maybe you can infuse the memory of chocolate with the sadness and disappointment you felt when you ate it. Then chocolate won't be a reward, it will be a reminder of the worst times. It's worth a try...

We are up against a barrage of advertising and food messages that try to persuade us that the processed versions are the most idyllic, the ones guaranteed to induce happiness.

So it might be time to invent our own story, one where fruit and vegetables take centre stage, and make us feel good. Because if you try them, and notice how great your body is when it's fuelled by natural foods, you might just rewrite your script.

Chocolate

Do you prefer dark or milk? Or perhaps white (yes, that's still chocolate...). Would you prefer a bar of it, or would you rather a box of Maltesers, or chocolate almonds? When do you crave it most?

Chocolate has become a phenomenon in our society. Revered, feared, desired....Chocolate is listed as the most craved food by women. It is cited as the secret indulgence. It is given as romantic gifts. Bought as consolation. Eaten as a treat, a reward, a condolence. It is blamed for weight gain, obesity and broken diets.

Does it really deserve this? After all, isn't chocolate just another food?

Having worked for Cadbury for five years, I have a large personal experience with chocolate. I once dug out a bath tub full of solid chocolate: molten chocolate was wheeled around the factory in these tubs in cases of emergency (and no – pre-menstrual cravings didn't count as an emergency). In this instance, the chocolate had solidified and the only way to get it out was to dig it out with a shovel. It was just like digging the garden. Big spadefuls of heavy brown gloop.

Crazy Diets: Patricia Highsmith

Novelist Patricia Highsmith ate the same thing for virtually every meal: bacon and fried eggs.

She began each writing session with a stiff drink – "not to perk her up", according to her biographer, Andrew Wilson, "but to reduce her energy levels, which veered towards the manic".

Then she would sit on her bed surrounded by cigarettes, coffee, a doughnut and a saucer of sugar, the intention being "to avoid any sense of discipline and make the act of writing as pleasurable as possible".

I have also eaten a huge amount of chocolate. Working for Cadbury, I was surrounded by it and some days I ate little else. I actually worked in a chocolate factory for almost a year. Everyone told me that after the first few weeks I would stop eating chocolate. In fact, the reverse happened. After the first few weeks, I stopped eating all other food, and just lived off the chocolate in the factory. The shift work (I was running the Crunchie plant, if you really want to know) didn't suit me, and I felt permanently jet-lagged and slightly unwell. The combination of the lack of sleep and the appalling diet meant I put on an awful lot of weight, very fast.

When I stopped working for Cadbury it was a long time before I could stomach chocolate again. That might sound hard to believe. After all, I was the person who, at four in the morning, was hiding in the factory, cramming broken pieces of chocolate into my mouth as if there was no tomorrow.

I still eat chocolate, although not in the same quantity that I did back then, and certainly not to the exclusion of everything else.

If you can learn anything from my mistakes (and the whole point of this book is to try to save you the trouble that I had, losing weight) it is this: if you would eat your own body weight in chocolate, given half the chance, don't go and work in a chocolate factory.

Chocolate is an intensely pleasurable thing to eat. Any food that has a melting point just lower than our body temperature has a delightful feel on the tongue. The cocoa butter in chocolate melts at 30C into a molten, sweet liquid in the mouth.

Research shows that fat, sugar, texture and aroma, combine in chocolate to create a hedonic (or pleasure) response that can generate cravings similar to drugs or alcohol. Science has also shown chocolate to contain several psychoactive ingredients that can cause psychological or behavioural change that parallel other addictive substances, theobromine being one of these. Theobromine acts on the body in a similar manner to caffeine, and adds weight to the conclusion is that cravings are real, and that chocolate has a genuine effect on our biology.

While that might explain why we like it, and why we crave it, it can't be blamed for obesity. If you ate a bar of chocolate every day as part of your balanced diet, and as part of your daily intake (not additional to) then you would not become fat. It might not be the healthiest way to eat, but it is a perfectly legitimate way to eat.

If you sneak a large bar of Dairy Milk every night on the way home from work, then you are very likely to put on weight. Remember Michael, who every day, on the way back from work, he bought a kilogram of Dairy Milk, and ate it in the car. If you eat chocolate like that, have a bar every day in addition to your daily food needs, cram it in without tasting... then you are likely to put on weight.

If you love chocolate, have it. Have it every day if you want! But plan to have it. Enjoy it. Savour it.

And you never know, if you have enough of it, you may tire of it.

Can't I get slim on junk food?

An American professor of nutrition has, in the name of research, spent ten weeks losing weight on junk food. He wanted to prove that it could be done. And it has been done! He has spent weeks on a diet of biscuits, cakes and other high-sugar, fat-laden junk food and has generated a great deal of media hype with tales of weight loss, deeper sleep and better general health.

Mark Haub is an associate professor from the department of human nutrition at Kansas State University. Over ten weeks, Mark ate sponge cakes, biscuits, some raw vegetables and drank full fat milk and a protein shake every day. He lost 12.1 kilograms from his original 91.3-kilogram body weight.

The but (and it's a big one) is that he carefully controlled his calories intake. He limited his intake to a maximum of 1800 calories (7531 kilojoules) a day, exercised heavily throughout the period and took vitamin supplements in addition to "muscle" protein shakes.

At one point he estimated that he had worked off, and not replaced, more than 800 calories through an abnormally strenuous workout.

"I am not recommending or promoting this approach. I am simply in the process of illustrating that foods deemed to wreck diets, cause obesity, lead to diabetes, etc... do not - in and of themselves - do that," he said after four days and a 3.2-kilogram loss.

On September 10, he ate:

- a double espresso
- two servings of Hostess Twinkies Golden Sponge Cake
- one Centrum Advance Formula "From A To Zinc" pill
- one serving of Little Debbie Star Crunch cookies
- a Diet Mr Dew drink
- half a serving of Doritos Cool Ranch corn chips
- two servings of Kellogg's Corn Pops cereal
- a serving of whole milk
- half a serving of raw baby carrots
- one and a half servings of Duncan Hines Family Style Chewy Fudge brownie
- half a serving of Little Debbie Zebra Cake
- one serving of Muscle Milk Protein Shake drink
- Total: 1589 calories

He has shown that you can eat chocolate, biscuits and lose weight. The secret lies in the quantity or portion size.

If you love a particular fast food, there is no reason to eliminate it from your diet. In fact, it would be better for you to include it on a regular and moderate basis, rather than binge on it intermittently.

Mark proved (in a one-man experiment) that one biscuit doesn't break a diet. In fact, it can be the foundation for a diet, albeit a not-very-healthy one. He proved that weight loss doesn't have to ban foods. You can lose weight and still include all kinds of treats that aren't usually associated with dieting.

Despite the poor quality of his diet, his health improved over the ten week period. His blood pressure went down and various other measures improved. The health benefits of his weight loss outweighed the poor nutritional quality of his diet. That's not a message that we hear very often. Perhaps it's a concept that might be useful if you need to lose weight. It can be very freeing to know that it doesn't really matter what you eat, you can still shed the kilos as long as calories are reduced.

There would be other challenges, if you subsist entirely on processed food. It can be addictive, which would make it hard to limit portions and quantity. It wouldn't be a nutritious way to live, or particularly good for your long term health. However, if you really want to?

The answer is yes - you can get slim on junk food.

ACTION

If you choose, you can lose weight on junk food. Decide if that's right for you.

How much junk food do you really want to eat. Is it appealing to include it in your regular eating habit?

Childhood Memories. Or 'I blame my family'

"Dad used to take us to McDonalds on the weekend. We never saw him in the week, not after he and Mum split up, so it was a real treat. We could eat exactly what we wanted, no rules, no 'having to eat your greens'. I remember slurping on that milkshake, all thick and cool and creamy, until my head felt like it was gripped by an icy hand. Then those burgers, and the toys. The problem is, when I drive past McDonalds now, I still feel a little urge to go in. It's like having a bit of a hug from Dad. I miss him. And sometimes that's the closest I can get."

Peter, 37

Maria remembers the first time she went back to her parent's home town in Italy. She was sitting on a hot stone wall eating the most sublime ice cream she'd ever tasted, something that was a rare treat for her in those days, as her mother was always pressurising her about her weight. Linda remembers the birthday cakes her mother used to bake, licking out the bowls, her fingers sticky with cake mixture and then icing as her Mum cooked. These are special memories of happy times, and they often involve food. Chocolate is given as gifts, chips are bought late at night as a treat, or as a small child, perhaps you remember crisps stolen from tables at parties. Special memories aren't created around lettuce and apples. No one takes their children out for carrots.

Strawberries have a place close to my heart as one of our treats as children was going strawberry picking. You could only do it for about a month a year, and there was a strange delight in collecting a punnet full of red berries. I am partial to strawberries, in a way that I am not to raspberries. If I compare them, I prefer the taste of raspberries. But there is a memory attached to strawberries, an association with summer days, and heavy punnets of fruit and cream that is unbreakable.

Many parents reward their children with food. Whether it's a jelly bean as a small child for eating our vegetables, or a chocolate bar as a teenager for tidying our room, it is a common way of recognising achievements. It can be, therefore, a way that we reward ourselves for tasks completed, or hard days at work.

Shirley used to go out for chips with her Dad on a Friday night, and the memory of that means she turns to them in times of need. "I deserve some hot chips," says Shirley, "Every time I meet with my boss, I feel exhausted. I prepare for the meeting, he always asks difficult questions, and he never says well done. If I buy myself hot chips, sprinkled with salt, the crunch melting into the fluffy potato in the middle, at least I've had a reward. I feel like I'm recognised for a job well done."

As someone once said "You're not a dog. You don't need dog biscuits as a reward." The problem is, we have a psychology that is remarkably similar to dogs, and such rewards work astonishingly well. Just not for our waistlines.

It's not only reward that food can be used for in families. It can be a battlefield. When I was growing up, my parents told me to clean my plate. I was berated about the poor children starving in other countries. However long it took, I had to sit at the table until my plate was empty. I hated meat, and those roast pork dinners would take me forever to finish, until I cut the meat into tiny pieces and swallowed each morsel with a glass of water like a pill.

I still have a problem with leaving things on my plate, even if I had absolutely no say in how much was put there. (Sometimes I wonder how far I would take it? If you put kilograms of food on my plate, how much would I struggle through before I gave up?) Many of us accept what we are served without question, and yet as serving sizes are becoming larger and larger, its worth thinking about how much is enough.

Even though I know it's a decades-old message about clearing my plate, and isn't logical, I still find it hard to break.

Maria's Italian heritage equates food to love, and her relatives insist that you are lavished with food, and that you eat everything you're offered if you are to be part of the family. That's a pretty tough thing to do if you're trying to lose weight or look after your health.

Families and parents create all kinds of messages around food, dieting and bodies. These messages seep into our unconscious without our noticing because they have surrounded us since we were born. It takes a lot of work and courage to notice them, and even more to question them.

They are often behind some of the beliefs and rules that we have around food, beliefs and rules that aren't always helpful. It's possible to move on from these beliefs, and it's possible to have memories associated with food and not act on them. The more we acknowledge what they might be, then the more we can work with them.

It can be worth exploring the belief, messages and rituals that you were exposed to growing up. They may have been different in your immediate family compared to your extended family. There may have been experiences that were particularly formative. Perhaps whole food groups were not part of it. I have a friend who had never tried blue cheese until he was in his twenties, something that amazed me, as my family ate loads of it. One of my closest friends at university had been raised in a household with no chocolate. As a result neither he nor his sister got what all the fuss was about.

It's the emotional content around food that tends to be more pervasive. The pressures to eat or not eat, to clear the plate, or to eat Nanna's dessert. These can last a lifetime, and affect our attitudes to food more than we realise.

ACTION

What parental messages were there in your family around food and eating? Write some of them down and ask if they still apply to you now that you are an adult.

Were there emotional games or pressure around food consumption and meal times?

Do you have pleasant memories of certain foods that are associated with family memories? Does that make you crave them when you need comfort?

Calorie counting: maths was never my strong point

Everyone knows that to lose weight, you have to burn more calories than you take in. Well, almost everyone.

This has been scientifically proven time and again. It is a simple equation. Energy in minus energy out equal weight loss or gain. It's actually based on physics: thermodynamics. Our bodies are 'closed systems'. Which means any energy that goes in (in the form of calories) can only be used up or stored (as fat). It doesn't matter what form this 'energy' takes - even if it's kale and goji berries. Eating more than your system needs, will result in the excess being stored. As fat. There is no other option.

So in theory, if you knew how many calories you burned you could calculate how many calories you needed to eat to lose weight. And this is where it all falls down. How on earth would you know how many calories you burn?

There are all kinds of weight and height charts that can estimate these for you. For my height, these charts tell me I burn 1800 calories a day. That's quite a lot. However, closer examination and a few conversations with medical professional later, I was given an admission that in actual fact, I could burn as few as 1000 a day - depending on circumstances. Now that seems like a pretty large leeway for error to me....

The reason that its so hard to know how many calories we each burn is that it depends on many factors including:

Our lean muscle mass

i.e. how much of my body is muscle, compared to fat or water. Muscles burn calories even when resting so increasing your muscle mass is one of the easiest ways to raise your metabolic rate. Every additional kilogram of muscle burns more calories

Our activity throughout the day

Activity burns calories through movement – walking, running, gardening, cleaning – any activity increases energy usage

How often we eat

Research has shown that the very act of eating stimulates the metabolism – somehow the body recognises that more fuel is arriving, it digests it and gets ready to burn it. Therefore eating smaller more regular meals can assist in calorific usage

Our hormones

Different hormones can affect metabolism – for example testosterone encourages the building of muscles and therefore increases metabolism, whereas insulin has been shown to be linked to the laying down of fat stores

Our genetic make-up

Genetics can establish slight differences in metabolic rate

A full body scan (such as a Dexa scan) is one of the most accurate ways of measuring body composition, and this might give us a more reasonable estimate of our calorific needs. But even with that information, on any given day I might burn anything between 1000 and 2000 calories – it is anyone's guess.

There is only one source that can accurately calculate how many calories a day I burn. And that is my body. It has a built-in communication system to tell me how many it's using. It's the hunger mechanism: hunger kicks in when the body needs more fuel.

This means that while the logic of calories counting is sound, putting it into practice so that it works, can be tricky, and so far we have only tried to work out what we are burning off.

Then come the task of counting the calories of what you put into your mouth. A chart may say a small apple has 40 calories. How small is small? Everything is getting bigger these days... a spoonful of sugar has 16 calories – well – what sized spoon? Heaped or flat? It is impossible to be accurate. Unless everything you eat is weighed and measured accurately, it is nigh on impossible to calculate the calories eaten each day. Besides which, most of us forget the majority of what we eat, or fail to include the calories we drink. In fact, we're already seen that studies show that most people severely underestimate the amount they eat each day. (see the chapter on recording what we eat).

Calorie counting is therefore highly flawed as you can think you are doing a great job of counting them, when you really have no idea of whether you are burning these up or not or whether you are counting them accurately or not. Besides which, it is a huge effort to calculate everything that you put in your mouth, particularly when the food or meal has been prepared by someone else.

It is a well established fact that people do not accurately record their food intake when asked to. No prizes for guessing: people underestimate the amount of calories they eat. The degree of underreporting can be quite severe. One study compared twins where one was obese and the other was not. Both twins under-reported their intake, but the obese twin under-reported by an average of 764 calories per day more.

Another study found some individuals to be under-estimating their food intake by as much as 2000 calories per day. That's more than most of us are supposed to eat in a day!

In fact, paying people doesn't help them record their intake more accurately. The error in reporting is still huge. And neither does monitoring what they actually eat: people will still underreport even when they know their calorie intake can be verified.

In one ultra-embarrassing study, they ran the same experiment with dieticians. Even the professionals, the dieticians themselves, under-report their food intake: not quite as badly as the majority of us, but they still record less than they actually eat.

It's easy to see that we might simply fail to report all of the food we eat, misreport the portion sizes, or incorrectly describe the foods. Or perhaps we can't be bothered; the task of recording food intake can be quite tedious and we might not be diligent in weighing and recording all foods.

But the truth is more insidious. Even if the diary is only for our own eyes, we still don't stick to the truth. Snacks are missed off, that bite you had from your spouse's doughnut - that doesn't count and isn't recorded. The taste of cheesecake at the office party - no need to write that down.

Many of us swear that we don't eat a lot of calories but struggle to lose weight. But if most of us are this inaccurate in assessing how much we are really eating, then it's going to be hard to know why or how the kilos are mounting up. No wonder most of us say "But I hardly eat anything - I've no idea why my jeans don't fit."

In a hilarious, but quite embarrassing twist, one cunning researcher decided to supply overweight people with the amount of calories they claimed to be eating according to their food diaries. For example, a women who claimed to be eating 1200 calories per day was supplied with that actual amount of food. What happened? She lost 1.7 pounds per week.

One of the painful truths that we might have to face about ourselves is that we might eat more than we think. It can be useful to track what you eat for a week, but only if that doesn't bring up too many memories of diets, and make you want to cheat even more (it may have that effect). It can be an interesting exercise to see what you really eat and when.

So let's look at more useful and sustainable ways of living our lives and managing our weight. Weighing and measuring everything in minute detail is not sustainable.

The only way that calories are useful, are as a guide to roughly how much energy one food source contains compared to another. However – I'm sure your body will tell you that it can walk further on a chocolate than it can on cucumber.

If you're really struggling with how much you should be eating, a calorie count can be a good starting point. But the best starting point is your body's natural hunger mechanism. If you can get off the insulin rollercoaster, by eating regular protein, and not too much highly processed carbohydrate, then it will tell you when it needs feeding. You may find it disappointing how rare it is for you to be truly hungry.

ACTION

Stop counting calories and start listening to when your body really needs food

Summary

It doesn't really matter whether you like celery or burgers, chocolate or chips, you can lose weight and you can become more healthy.

A lower body weight is a great predictor of good health, however you get there. I'm not recommending a diet of junk food. I'm just suggesting that what you eat is your choice and all choices are valid.

Your food preferences are completely individual. Listen to your body, listen to what you want to eat.

And then enjoy it.

CHAPTER SEVEN
SOCIAL REASONS

Eating is a social activity, and for this reason, social pressures can undo many of the best intentions.

Friends encourage us to have another drink, or a slice of cake. The temptations at a restaurant prove too much to bear.

We're left with the choice of either being a hermit, living in isolation so that we can pursue our health goals, or undoing the good work of a week in a single meal on a Friday night.

It is possible to have a social life without finding yourself alternatively gorging and then starving to undo the damage.

It's a holiday or feast day! Diets start the day after.

Every time Maria celebrates Christmas with her family, she swears it will be different. She promises herself that she won't overeat, that she will resist the brandy butter, that she'll stop eating mince pies on the sofa when she's already stuffed. But the minute she walks into her parents' house, with its familiar, worn parquet floor, and the faded floral wallpaper, something in her switches. It's almost like she's a teenager again.

Her mother's enquiries about her job grate on her, because she knows that her mother really thinks she should be shooting kids out of her nether regions in a rapid volley of child-bullets. It's only feigned interest, heavy with emotional blackmail, and usually followed with: "Did I tell you that Gloria is going to be a grandmother for the SECOND time next year?"

Maria reaches for the homemade parmesan grissini (breadsticks) before she's been inside for ten minutes. An hour later, while her father prepares to carve the turkey, she's standing in the larder, spooning brandy butter into her mouth straight from the dish, the sweet, boozey buttery confection melting on her on tongue and sweetening the bitterness she feels inside.

Greta, meanwhile, slinks into her family home, her willpower battened down with iron rods. She will not touch the chocolates. She will not eat the mince pies. The day becomes a dance between her mother pushing food on her, and her refusal. Tension simmers. Her brother teases her about being on a diet. Her father pleads with her just to have a taste. Anger rises in her and the fury only serves to make her more determined.

For some of us, Christmas, Easter, birthdays, weddings are glorious days, days of celebration, feating, family and friends. These times are special, so we tell ourselves that we can't possibly stick to a diet. It's a reason to gorge on the many treats on offer: roast turkey with all the trimmings, Christmas pudding with brandy butter and cream, marzipan, mince pies and chocolate. We are then left with a sinking feeling and the repercussions of overeating. For some, this starts with the first mouthful. Others stave off the guilt until the celebrations are over and the ramifications of all that food are evident in the mirror.

Many years ago, when food was expensive and scarce, Christmas was a rare treat. These days, it's just another in a long line of celebrations, and our waistlines bear witness to this. Perhaps we don't need to gorge ourselves - perhaps there is a middle road?

We may feel crushed by the pressure from well meaning relatives to either eat more, or go on a diet. Perhaps we are flayed by the comments on our appearance, some well-meaning, and others downright cruel: Haven't you lost weight? Aren't you looking well? Or: what have you been doing to yourself? It may seem that the best way to cope with it all is several large meals, lots of alcohol and a few boxes of chocolate in between. And how else to recover than with the promise of another diet.

This is no way to celebrate. These occasions needs a whole new approach if we are to really enjoy them.

One such approach is to make a conscious decision about how we are going to eat, before we arrive at the event or day. This isn't a decision about what you are going to eat, or how much. It isn't a straightjacket. It is a decision about the way in which you are going to approach eating. Remind yourself that food is to be enjoyed, not rushed. Remind yourself that you can enjoy yourself in other ways than with food.

It can be helpful to remember that, most likely, this will not be your last wedding or Christmas or whatever on this earth. (I hope not.) So perhaps you don't have to eat everything on offer - there will be other opportunities to eat this kind of food. You might decide to eat those things that you really enjoy, and to leave everything else. Why eat the meat or the vegetables if what you really want is the dessert? Don't eat the dessert if you crave the cheese. Or have tiny bits of everything if you just want to sample.

If the food is important to you, concentrate on really enjoying every mouthful. Mindless eating while you're talking will have several pounds accumulate around your waist before you know it. Savour the food, relish it. Discuss it with your neighbour. And if it disappoints, register that you are disappointed, and don't just eat it anyway, push it to one side and promise yourself something nicer later. If the cake isn't up to scratch, promise to bake yourself a nicer one on the weekend. If the meat is tough, don't force it down.

If awkward relatives are like a sour sauce on the entire meal, it can be helpful to have a couple of comments on reserve. It doesn't matter whether you are worried that people will comment on your appearance or other aspects of your life. Such comments can be disconcerting whether positive or negative. A "Wow - you've lost weight" can have as many psychological ramifications as a "Gosh, you're heavier". The feeling of pressure to conform or maintain a weight or appearance can be great. Instead, practice saying something that you can use to most comments such as "I'd prefer you not to comment on my weight" or "The most important things happen to people on the inside". This way, at least you can feel prepared and you never know, it may ward off comments at the next gathering.

Relatives may also pressure you to eat food that you don't really want to eat "But I cooked this especially for you". "It's my speciality, you must try it". A polite 'no thank you' will suffice. You don't need to explain yourself. You can smile while you say it, and accompany it with an expression of love or appreciation for that person "you always make such an effort, but really, no thank you". Learn to stand up for what is right for you.

Sometimes I'm grateful not for Christmas, but for the fact that it only comes once a year.

Crazy Diets: Princess Diana's trick

Princess Diana's guests never knew she was eating the low fat version of their food.

Her former chef says: "She used to trick people: She'd say, 'Make me a mousse for President Reagan.' She couldn't have it because there was mayonnaise and sour cream. So she'd say 'Make me a fat-free version.' So I did. Often, when guests would come, she'd have the fat-free version and the guests were on the full-fat version and no one would know the difference."

(How would you feel if your friend cooked something high calories for you, while she smugly ate their way through a healthy version? True friends support you in your health and weight goals, and the whole underhand approach to this strikes chills through me. At the very least she could have offered her guests the choice of either the full or the low fat version.)

Because you can't eat out and stay slim

I arrive at the restaurant and look at the menu. I can't quite concentrate on the conversation until I've decided what to eat. Burger and chips. I definitely shouldn't have that. My eye keeps wandering back to it. A salad, that's what I should have - a Caesar Salad.

"I think I'll have a Caesar salad," I say

"You do know that's got more fat in it than a burger..." says Colin.

Has it? I don't want the salad then. I can't have the burger. I don't want to get fat. A creamy pasta dish catches my eye. No, no cream.

Someone is saying my name.

"Didn't you have an important meeting this week?" they are asking.

I can't focus on that. What should I eat?

Going out to eat might be an opportunity to let loose and throw off the dieting chains. Or it might be a terrifying event where you can't bear to veer off the diet even slightly, for fear that you'll never get back on the straight and narrow.

Sometimes you don't get a say and other people order for the table, choosing your food for you. Other times you have to share food from joint plates and you don't know if you are going to get enough.

"If I'm going out to eat, even if it's a business lunch," says Andrea, "I'll try to starve myself that morning or the whole day, because I'm so worried about the calories in the lunch or dinner. I'll start worrying about it days before, it's ridiculous. I know its something I should be looking forward to but instead I'm panicking about how much I'll eat. I'll keep telling myself that I won't eat much, that I'll just push it around my plate (which I never do - I see some women do that and I wonder how).

"And then the worst thing is, on my way to the lunch, or the dinner, I'll stop and buy a huge bag of Maltesers. A massive one, and I'll eat them as fast as I can, telling myself again and again how little I'll eat at the meal out. Then, of course, when I get to the restaurant, I'm not hungry, and I don't eat very much. But it would have been far more enjoyable, and probably far less fattening for me to just eat the lunch or dinner, and not had the Maltesers. Why am I so ridiculous?"

When you go out to a restaurant, you get to choose what you eat. At someone else's home, you are at their mercy. If they have cooked potatoes slathered in butter, or a rich pastry pie, you may feel your good intentions crumble.

Some resort to fictitious food allergies to get out of eating food that they fear will make them fat.

Going out to eat, whether at a restaurant or at someone's house, is a time to go back to basics. Give yourself permission to eat what you really feel like, without rules around what you can and can't have. Take time to enjoy the food and try to stop when you've had enough, which may be before your plate is empty. This means checking on yourself to see when your hunger has abated.

If you're not hungry, choose a starter. If you don't like the look of the main courses, or find that all too much, you can always opt for two starters, one after the other. I love this, as I'm never tempted by the huge lump of meat that often constitutes the main dishes.

At other people's houses, we have less control. If you're trying to watch your weight, and the hostess serves up a dish smothered in cream, you may find your heart sinking. You know that after one mouthful you won't be able to resist eating the rest. If you find yourself in these situations, you always have a number of options available to you. One is to have a quiet word with the hostess, explain that you are trying to eat less, or watching your weight, or whatever feels comfortable. You can ask for a small portion. You can accept that it might not be your choice to eat it, but that you'll have a small amount and really enjoy it.

Whatever you decide, don't beat yourself up if you eat more than you intended. That's normal. We all do it. It doesn't mean that you have to starve yourself. You may find it means you're less hungry the following day, in which case, work with that and eat a little less.

ACTION

When eating out, try to stay in tune with your body and eat what will make you satisfied.

Try not to eat beyond the point of fullness.

Summary

Holidays such as Christmas and Thanksgiving can put a huge amount of pressure on us to eat. Even if we don't feel pressure to eat, there is a lot of temptation, and the prospect of ending the celebrations heavier and less healthy than we might choose.

Make a conscious decision before events on how you are going to approach them. Try not to starve yourself, or wreck your blood sugar before you even get there and if you do end up eating more than you wanted to, try to be gentle with yourself.

Plan a few things to say to awkward relatives, if that helps you deal with unfortunate comments that might come your way.

If you're going out to eat, take your time to work out what you'd really like to eat, and then make sure you enjoy it.

Crazy diets: William the Conqueror's booze diet

The first recorded diet was for William the Conqueror in England. He got so podgy that he couldn't ride a horse. As horses were the major mode of transport at the time, this was quite a drawback.

In order to lose weight, he adopted a liquid diet. The only liquid available at the time was alcohol (water wasn't safe to drink until the last century) so he must have been in a drunken stupor for most of his diet. Which lasted the best part of a year.

Things didn't end well. The next recorded event is his death. This was from falling off a horse. Whether this was because he was too drunk to stay on it, too fat for the horse, or now thin enough but hungover, we'll never know...

(So maybe you can get thin on the grog, but this strikes me as a little extreme.)

CHAPTER EIGHT
EMOTIONAL CUES

We are emotional beings, despite our rational minds. Psychology shows that most decisions are made on an emotional basis and then justified after the fact with 'rational' explanations.

Despite our ability to pull a reason for our behaviour out of the air, to rationalise it even if it isn't the true reason behind our behaviour, our underlying emotions exert a strong force, one that is hard to resist.

Eating or not eating, dieting or gaining weight or breaking our eating plans can unleash a maelstrom of emotions that then lead to disaster.

We don't have to be the slave to this. We can find a different way.

I feel bad about what I ate

It's too late now. I've eaten it all. My stomach is bloated, too full and swollen for my clothes. I loosen the buttons, undo my belt. I feel thirsty but if I drink, my abdomen feels as though it might burst.

There is something worse than the physical symptoms, worse than the bloating and the discomfort. I can feel emotions rising from the back of my throat, almost as though I'm vomiting up the tears, the self-hatred, the deep regret. Why did I eat so much? I was being so good. I had it under control. And now I've ruined it all. My body is fat and ugly again. I'm such a failure.

A wave of self-loathing crashes over me, and a small belch of

It's strange, isn't it, that you might eat even more when you're full, but that's exactly what scientists have found that dieters do. Non dieters, don't do that: the more you feed them, the less they eat. Dieters? They do the opposite. The fuller they get, the more they eat. If they think they've broken their diet, they eat even more.

About 40 years ago, a landmark study asked dieters and non-dieters to participate in what was billed as an ice cream tasting. Their only role was to rate the ice creams. They were given either one milkshake "pre-load", two milkshakes pre-load or nothing, prior to the tasting. They were then told to eat as much ice cream as they wanted or needed in order to rate them. The assumption was that the more milkshakes you consume before the tasting, the less you'll eat (because you're already full, right?).

The researchers found that those who were on strict diets actually ate MORE ice cream the more milkshakes they had beforehand. If dieters had one milkshake, that ate more than those dieters who were fed nothing. Those who drank two milk shakes, ate the most ice cream of all. The non-dieters did the opposite. The more full they were of milk shake, the less ice cream they ate.

The researchers hypothesised that dieters who constantly restrain their intake tend to become "disinhibited" after they break their diet boundary (sometimes referred to as the "what the hell" effect). This is the opposite of how our bodies are supposed to work. The more we eat, the less we are supposed to want.

All of this supposes that we aren't constantly in a state of deprivation due to food restriction. It assumes that we haven't created a 'world of scarcity', where we never feel as if we have enough, where we never really know when the next meal is coming from, and whether or not we are going to enjoy it.

Perhaps you recognise something of yourself in this scenario. It was certainly true of me when I was trying to lose weight, to the extent that just eating too much at a meal could trigger me to eat more. The actual sensation of being overly full led me to eat more. Partly because I felt guilty for allowing myself to be uncomfortable, partly through despair at losing weight.

Whatever the reason, it's something to be aware of. If being overly full triggers you to eat more, then try to avoid that if you can. If you find yourself wanting to eat more because you either feel that you've 'blown it' or because your stomach is uncomfortable after a meal, then try to talk yourself down from the ledge. It doesn't need to be the starting point for more eating.

You just ate a little too much. It wasn't a crime. It's not permanent. Your body will digest the food. Try to relax and remember what you enjoyed about the meal you had. If you find yourself struggling to stop eating, go back to the chapter on fullness and satisfaction.

ACTION

If you feel bad about what you ate, consider the research that shows you are likely to eat more, even while you are still uncomfortably full.

Try to remember that you haven't overeaten because you are bad or weak. You are human, and the tendency to do things to excess, particularly things that are bad for us, seems to be an illogical, but common trait of all of us.

The perils and pitfalls of snacking.

I've just sat down again having wandered into the kitchen – looked at the biscuits, gazed at nuts and searched for something. Something to ease the slight discomfort I feel in myself at the moment. I'm almost properly hungry, just starting to get there. I'm also a bit stuck with work and don't want to struggle through those problems.

Snacking and nibbling can cure so many ills: anxiety, restlessness, impatience, anger. Nibble nibble nibble like a little mouse. A biscuit here, a sweet there. A piece of chocolate, someone else's leftovers. Nibble nibble. A few crisps or nuts, and maybe, yes, another handful of those. And before you know it, you've eaten your whole day's calories without even noticing.

That is the main problem with snacking and nibbling. You don't really notice. A handful of dry cereal from the packet. A corner of cheese. A spoonful of ice cream.

You'd notice if you'd sat down at a table and had eaten a bowl of cereal with milk, or a cheese sandwich. You would have felt nourished, full, overfull even. But nibbling isn't really about feeding yourself and nurturing yourself. It's eating without eating. Consumption that doesn't count. It's hoping to bypass boredom or time or uncomfortable emotions without actually getting fat.

Eating without noticing is one of the fastest ways to put on weight.

Snacks are so easy to forget. They are usually high calories and not very filling. In fact some (like a handful of sugary lollies or sweets) can even make you feel hungrier shortly afterwards. If you want a snack, try and get a plate, and make a proper small meal.

I can feel you resisting. "But then I'll get fat if I eat all that." "But I don't want a proper meal'. If you don't want a proper meal, perhaps you're not hungry and you actually don't need a snack either. In the event that you are hungry, maybe it would be better that you register that you've eaten something, something substantial, which might sustain you and prevent you from nibbling again in half an hour.

There are other hazards of snacking. The constant stimulation of our stomach means that it never has a chance to rest, or more importantly 'clean up'. We have brilliant little helpers in our guts that maintain our bodies. If we have eaten a steak, it might take five hours for it to be digested in the stomach and small intestine. Once this is done, the small intestine sweeps itself in a such a cute manner that even tough-minded scientists have called it the 'housekeeper'. If we eat before it has a chance to do this, it once again goes on standby to receive food. But constant snacking means there is no time for 'cleaning' which helps keep our gut healthy.

The drip feed of food also keeps insulin churning up and down. Our bodies don't have an opportunity to find their point of homeostasis where blood sugar and hormones are regulated, balanced and consistent and don't have to deal with a constant influx of food. This constant demand for insulin, to deal with the food, can artificially inflate our appetite. So constant nibbling and snacking not only adds to our waistline because we're not paying attention to it, but also because it makes us want to eat more.

If you find yourself snacking and nibbling, ask yourself whether you feel hungry, or whether it is something else that is driving you to the food source. If you are hungry, put something on a plate and focus on it and if you're not, try to work out what else you might need.

ACTION
Snacks are a very recent invention. Do you find them helpful, or are they an excuse to extend eating until it lasts most of the day?

You hate your thighs

"I hate my thighs"
"If only my stomach was flatter"
"I can't stand my bum"

Ask a woman about her body, and what she thinks of it and she'll most likely say "I hate my....." Get any woman to look in the mirror and it's unlikely she'll see a goddess looking back at her. Instead she'll see a list of flaws and imperfections. Interestingly, I have seen many a man strut up and down in front of a glass, ignorant of the beer belly and balding pate, stroking himself and admiring his physique. I fear this is changing with the pressure on men to have six-packs and biceps like Thor, but there is something endearing about a chap who thinks he looks rather fab. I wish more of us could be like that.

Instead, we are filled with hatred and disgust about our bodies. Sometimes hatred is combined with anger or a sense of injustice. We're supposed to be long-legged, high breasted, tanned, taut, lightly muscled, flat-stomached, lithe and beautiful young specimens. These are the pictures in the magazines, the stars in the movies, the aspirational images. We're bombarded with so many images of beautiful and perfect bodies, that we can't help but fall short with our wobbly, wrinkly, saggy, blotchy humanity.

In reality, we come in all shapes and sizes. Short legs, pot bellies, broad hips, hefty arms. Our necks are short, our skins wrinkle and burn. Our stomachs have borne children, our feet are blistered from crazy (but beautiful) shoes. We have tan lines and freckles, moles and birthmarks. Scars and injuries mark us - our histories written on our skin. Genetics and family traits are revealed in our eye colour, our height, the length of a neck or the shape of a leg. We are the sum of all that's gone before.

Yet the images that bombard us are ever more perfect. The art of airbrushing and photoshopping irons out anything viewed as less than perfect. Lighting and make-up camouflage more flaws, and as surgery removes any last imperfections it's no wonder that we all compare ourselves with these divine beauties and find ourselves falling a long way short

As Cindy Crawford once said: "Even I don't wake up looking like Cindy Crawford."

Eventually we start to resent this constant pressure and unrealistic expectation, and begin to crave those magazines that offer 'Celebrities with cellulite' or "stars without make-up'. We need some reminder that perhaps they are not as perfect as they look. Research has shown that women's self esteem diminishes after reading glossy magazines. These unreal images really do damage our views of ourselves.

Body hatred is not productive – it doesn't make the world a better place, or make marriages more content. In fact, I suspect it brings on bad moods (bad body days), worse sex (with the lights off or certain body parts off limits) and a general dissatisfaction with life.

Some might argue that we need to hate our bodies in order to change them. If we accept and love them, we might never lose weight. Maybe there is a fear that if we accept them then we will never change them - we will never lose the weight that we want to lose. And while our bodies are far more than what they look like, there are vast benefits to being a healthy weight.

Let me put it to you like this: imagine you have two children that you are to teach, for a year. The first child you shower with love and affection, telling them they are fabulous. The second child, you hate. You insult the child, and list their flaws endlessly.

Which child will have learned more and behaved better at the end of the year? The second child will be collapsed in a pool of despair, whereas the one you have loved and encouraged will be flourishing. Were you shocked to think of insulting and hating a child? Many of us think of our own bodies that way - hating them, insulting them. Imagine how would it be to treat someone else the way you treat your body, the way you think of your body? It's a sobering thought.

What if we were to accept the bodies we have? Perhaps it is not until we truly accept our bodies that we will be kind enough to nurture them into their best selves, into the glowing, gleaming curves of desire they were born to be?

Body love is such a key part of being kind and compassionate to ourselves. It doesn't mean convincing yourself that your legs are long and willowy when in truth they will only ever be short. It's about accepting that your legs are short. That might not have been your first choice, but that's what you got in the genetic lottery. And no amount of self hatred, dieting, self denial (or even cosmetic surgery, god forbid) will ever make them long and willowy.

It's then about dressing to flatter those legs, about making them short and cute instead. It's about loving them enough that you can laugh about them, flirt with them. And guys will fall for any woman who feels good enough about her body to flirt with it.

Some of us struggle to come to terms with the ravages of time, and believe me, time can be cruel. One woman described her belly, after childbirth, as jelly mauled by a tiger. Breasts (yes, even small ones) head southwards, lose the perkiness of youth.

We can choose to fight this, or we can enjoy the fact that we had better boobs once. And enjoy the fact that today, they look better now than they will in another ten years' time.

There is already a backlash in the media about the degree of manipulation that most photographs undergo, but that hasn't filtered down to how we feel about ourselves.

When you find yourself criticising or insulting or hating your body, try saying it aloud, but use your name. Such as 'I hate Clare's thighs, they're too fat'. Vocalising this, using your name in the third person can bring the thought into sharp focus. The cruelty of it is highlighted. Most of us would never say such a thing to another person.

Giving ourselves permission to feel good about ourselves, even if our bodies aren't perfect, also gives us permission to look after ourselves. It can really help us be kinder. It might sound counter-intuitive, but loving our imperfect, overweight bodies, will do more to resolve weight issues and over-eating, than a continuation of hatred, than the prolonging of a battleground where, let's face it, neither side wins.

ACTION

As critical thoughts of your body come to mind, write them down or vocalise them in the third person, using your name.

Write down the things that the body part you hate has done for you. Your thighs might walk you to work. Your stomach might digest your food or carry babies. Thank that part of your body, saying it aloud. How does that make you feel?

Do you feel compassion towards your body yet?

Summary

Just feeling bad about what we've eaten can compel us to eat more. In fact, sometimes the more full we feel, the more we eat.

It might be worth going back to the chapter on hunger and focusing on how your body feels, concentrating on what fullness feels like. Try not to be too hard on yourself if you've eaten too much. it is a well known trigger for eating more.

Snacking and nibbling may be recommended by some diets, but they can extend the eating period and overstimulate our stomachs and our bodies, making it harder to control our insulin levels and leaving our guts no time to clear up and heal themselves.

Finally, try to be kind to your wonderful body. It is capable of marvellous things.

CHAPTER NINE
WHEN YOU CAN'T STOP

Sometimes you just can't stop eating.

It can be a terrifying experience to feel so out of control. It can also be lonely, as most of us are too ashamed to admit to having done it, so then we feel both terrified and lonely. Anyone who hasn't done it will struggle to even understand it, to empathise. It seems impossible that a person might not be in control of their own actions, but a binge can feel like that.

This next section is about those times, which, if you can follow some of the guidelines in this book, will hopefully become fewer and fewer.

I binged

"Every time I think that one bite will be OK. I really believe that I'll be able to stop, but as soon as I've had one, I completely forget about stopping and I continue until I can hardly breathe for being so full.
Why can't I stick to the simple program? I keep thinking that I'm in control and I'm on a diet. But somehow I buy things out of habit and feelings of deprivation. As soon as I have a single taste, I completely forget about the program, about the diet. I lose control. And now I am slumped on on the kitchen floor, crying, I despair of every being slim.
Why can't I have my cake and eat it?"

Bella, aged 33

Research has shown that there is one main cause of bingeing. It is caused by dieting. Dieting increases the likelihood of developing an eating disorder by eighteen times. 1800 percent, not 18 percent. That is closer than the link between smoking and cancer.

Bingeing is the response of a body and mind that have been deprived and constrained for too long. We have not evolved to be in a state of deprivation. The body becomes imbalanced and hungers for either carbs, or fat, or whichever nutrients it needs. The body and mind seek those things of which they have been deprived. The mind becomes obsessed. Obsessed with whatever it cannot have and as you are 'not allowed' them, as soon as you have one taste, then the out of control bingeing starts.

Imagine that you will try to breathe only once every minute. Or that you will only sleep for three hours a night. Your body's needs will soon over-ride your so-called willpower. It will triumph and demand those things it needs – it will force you to breathe, to sleep. And yes – it will force you to eat.

I feel so sad that we fight our bodies so. I feel sad at how much I hated and despised my body and myself for not being able to stick to these impossible diets. I always felt that I was the failure for breaking the diet. I thought I didn't have the willpower or discipline. I thought it proved that I deserved to be overweight. I believed it meant I wasn't worthwhile. I thought I was the failure.

I didn't realise the diet was the failure. It was impossible to adhere to.

New research is showing that there may be a physical cause, and possible permanent damage from extreme dieting. The research we've reviewed in the section on fasting shows the same effects.

A binge is a craving for food, for sustenance, for nourishment. It is also a cry for love, for acceptance and for kindness.

ACTION

Think about a time in the past when you have binged and look at what was happening in your life before it. Had you been dieting? Were you feeling repressed or suppressed? Was your very being asking for something that you were not giving it?

What is a binge?

"Every bite is seasoned with loneliness, marinaded in pain. Each breath is stifled by the bloat in my stomach and the ache in my soul."

Maria, 55

A binge is any eating experience that does not feel in control, or conflicts with what or where you want to be. It can be anything from snatching a biscuit from a packet and hoping no one finds out, to eating 50,000 calories in any available form.

It might be stuffing a large bar of chocolate down in the car before you get home so no one can see. Sometimes it can involve sneaking leftovers from other's plates as you clear away. It might be taking food out of the garbage to fill that insatiable urge. Or it might be a three-week-long rampage of incessant eating until you feel you'll never come up for air.

A binge is usually accompanied by feelings of self-disgust and followed by a deep sense of guilt.

Often, during the binge, the eater becomes numb, almost in an altered state of consciousness. The world shrinks to the size of the mouth and the food that is going into it. The need becomes obsessive and the body goes onto auto-pilot, seemingly beyond any stop buttons or control. This only serves to increase the terrible feelings of guilt and horror when it is over.

It begins with an overwhelming hunger and need – usually after several days of strict dieting.

"I just need some real food, something to crunch, something to fill me up and give me some energy just for a little while. I think that maybe I'll just have one bran flake from the cereal packet – that won't be bad. I stand and open the packet and my heart starts racing. I shouldn't be doing this. But just one – it won't hurt. So I look and select the largest bran flake and crunch it. It tastes slightly sweet and satisfying and I can feel my blood racing to pick up the vital sugars it is delivering. Perhaps just one more, and I scan the contents of the box to find the next large one.

"Then, somehow, the world becomes dimmer and fainter, as I seek out another one. My focus shrinks to the contents of the cereal box. Reality vanishes and there is only my appetite. I stand in the kitchen, the pivot point of my life, seeking the best flakes and putting them in my mouth, totally absorbed. Somehow this process becomes automatic, rapid and I become hypnotised and mesmerised. Some time passes before I realise that I have consumed more than half a kilogram of Sultana Bran. Dry.

"The diet is clearly ruined. I feel bad. Worse than bad. I hate myself. The loathing rises in my gorge like vomit. I've wrecked it. Can't I stick at anything? I'll never lose weight this way. I don't even deserve to be thin, I'm so disgusting.

"Now I'll have to go on a really strict diet tomorrow because I've blown it today. I feel sick at my lack of control. I may as well have that chocolate. Especially as I'm not going to eat anything at all tomorrow.

"Later I find myself standing in the local shop. The choice overwhelms me. This is food I'm not allowed. Contraband. Forbidden treasure. The sweat of anxiety slicks of palms. I glance around. There's no one I know. No one recognises me. I buy several bars and rush out of the shop, tearing them open just outside and stuffing them into my mouth frantically, hoping that no one sees, not tasting them, swallowing quickly. My mouth is dry. I choke down another mouthful.

"Tears well up. How can I be so vile? Standing on a street corner stuffing my face. Now that I've sunk this low, I may as well have everything that I've been craving. All the forbidden foods that I've wanted over the weeks, all the things I've denied myself race into my brain unbidden. Ice cream, pastries, icing. And I gorge on them. Not tasting, just forcing it in. Eating while I can as I know tomorrow will be a harsh punishment indeed. An even sterner diet. I know how hungry I'm going to be, so I shove it all in now....."

Who can express the physical and psychological pain of a binge? Who can convey the self loathing and disgust that follows. The shame, the secrecy, the feelings of being out of control, isolated, hopeless. There is almost nothing worse we can do to ourselves.

It is the final cry for help from a psyche and body that is starved of nutrition, love, care and compassion.

It is the wretched act of desperation from a downtrodden, lonely, sad and ashamed human being. It is a cry for help.

How to stop a binge

I reckon this is pretty hard. I have read all kinds of tips, and if you are going to binge, most of these (varnishing your nails... taking a walk...) don't even begin to touch the overwhelming urge to obliterate everything. Anyone who thinks that varnishing your nails is going to stop the tidal wave of a binge has never been in the grip of one.

The pain preceding a binge can be so deep and so raw that we may not even recognise it. The urge to muffle the desperation and the anguish may skip our consciousness, as it's too awful to contemplate. This makes it hard to recognise the triggers, making it even harder to stop.

Sometimes the very early mouthfuls are the point at which we can interrupt. The point before all control has been lost, and where there is still some recognition of what is happening.

Calling or being with a close and understanding friend is the best thing I have found when the urge to binge strikes. This tends to provide the emotional succour that we are unable to provide for ourselves at that moment. Bingeing is a private and secretive activity, so whilst we might overeat with a friend, full scale bingeing is likely to stop, or at least be put on hold. It can be very hard to ask for help when you are feeling this low, particularly as you are likely to tell yourself that you should be able to control your food on your own.

Part of being kind to yourself, is to accept that, right at this moment, it is difficult and you are struggling. And if there is someone who can support you, then the best thing is to turn to them

However, on your way back home, the temptation may well return. (How many times have I driven into a garage and undone all the good my caring friend had done)

The easiest (and only long term) way to stop a binge is to stop dieting and to give up all lists of restricted or forbidden foods.

Even then, the experience of out-of-control eating may continue for some years, although in various guises. The length of a binge usually diminishes along with the quantity of food consumed, as dieting stops. It might become less and less extreme until eventually a binge is a few chocolates sneaked from a box when no-one was looking. But you, in yourself, still know it was a binge because of the shame, the secrecy and the feeling that you shouldn't be doing it. Even as the binges reduce in size and frequency they can still be distressing.

Even when you're in touch with your body and your hunger, even when your weight is at a point that you are happy, even then, painful issues will arise in your life. And these issues may make you question how you feel about yourself. At this point old behaviours and coping mechanisms may surface and you may find yourself turning to food. If you're not longer dieting and restricting your eating, these urges may be weaker, but they may still be there.

Be compassionate with yourself. Remember how far you have come. You have learned so much.

Recognise it for what it is: it is a cry for help. From either your body, which isn't getting the nutrition and food it needs. Or from your psyche, which is feeling deprived.

It might be worth revisiting whether you are being too harsh on yourself?

I don't know what to do after a binge

"I'm obsessing about slimming pills. I have gone completely crazy. It's the eating that causes the craziness. Overeating, especially sugar, makes me feel fat and then I obsess about diets, try to control my food intake by restricting it severely, and end up bingeing and then hate myself even more…
I want to turn to more and more extreme measures and it scares me. Slimming pills from the internet surely is a step too far?"
Laura, aged 44

After a binge you will, most likely, want to punish yourself. You may want to force a strict diet on yourself to rid yourself of the weight you have stuffed inside yourself. You may want to impose discipline on your unruly body by ramming it into a straitjacket of diet and exercise. You may want to give up all hope.

You may, like Laura, want to try more extreme methods. Drugs and slimming pills, laxatives and even vomiting. These are methods that lead to an even more slippery slope, a black pit that is really hard to pull yourself out of.

Try not to do this. Try to be kinder.

After a binge it will help greatly if you are able to be gentle and compassionate with yourself. You must have been feeling really terrible to do that to yourself. And you will be feeling worse now. So be kind to yourself. Forgive yourself. Don't try to punish yourself now or in the future with the promise of more restrictive diets, or rigorous exercise. These are actually further triggers that may extend the binge or cause another one.

Accept what has happened. Write down how you feel. Write down what else you could have done or how else you could have handled it. Call a friend. Be kind to yourself.

Promise yourself delicious food the next day. Assure yourself that you will eat only what you really want and enjoy, and that you will eat it as you need it, whatever the time is. Allow yourself to eat more of the 'forbidden' or binge foods if that is what you desire, but promise that you will serve them beautifully, and that you will eat them at a table.

Realise that your body and soul may feel battered and bruised. Sometimes literally. A large quantity of food can seriously hurt a stomach. And those who use laxatives or vomiting to try to purge the sensations of being over-stuffed will also suffer from those unnatural and cruel ways to treat our bodies.

You may look and feel bloated as your body will retain a lot of extra water to try to cope with the influx of food. Try to relax and know that your body will deal with this over the next few days and in a day or two, the bloating will have subsided.

Make sure you don't wear tight or restrictive clothing to punish yourself – tight waistbands will remind you cruelly of your stomach, that may be swollen after too much food. This kind of reminder will not teach you not to do it again. It will only make you feel bad. I remember putting on jeans that were too small, so that I could hardly walk, and hoping that they would miraculously compress my legs, or 'sweat' off the weight.

This is not a book about eating disorders. Signs that you might be suffering from one include vomiting, the use of laxatives, or a sense of being out of control. If you have an eating disorder, please contact a professional, or one of the eating disorder charities in your area for support. There are lots of places to go - please seek help if you need it.

Crazy Diets: Marlon Brando

Marlon Brando is famous for his weight problems, as much as his movie career.

He was known to eat peanut butter by the jarful, boxes of cinnamon buns and huge breakfasts consisting of cornflakes, sausages, eggs, bananas and cream, and pancakes drenched in maple syrup. He could devour up to six hotdogs at a time in late-night feasts.

If you tried to force him to diet, he would break refrigerator locks at night, flee film sets with giant tubs of ice-cream and enlist friends to throw burger bags over the gates of his Mulholland Drive estate.

CHAPTER TEN
EXCUSES, FALSE HOPES
AND THE REBEL WITHIN

Sometimes, we just don't want to face reality. We'd rather live in a world where nothing is our fault, where we don't have any responsibility.

Perhaps its a desire to return to childhood where we are looked after by others. We wish that our excuses are proven facts, that our bodies were to blame for their weight. We don't accept liability for anything, preferring to point the finger at our jobs, our stress levels or our love life.

It's natural to rebel against life - it can seem unfair, harsh and unrelenting. Sometimes, though, if we face reality, and look it square in the eyes, we can find a way through, a way that is easier than we might have thought.

Exercise: Surely that's an excuse to eat?

I remember as a child climbing trees with a sense of adventure, testing out my growing limbs, which grew stronger with each conquered tree. I rode my bike with friends, racing to see who won. I ran and walked, explored. I loved every minute of it and never considered it exercise. When did moving your body stop being fun?

Exercise can be a word synonymous with punishment. For many of us it summons images of unflattering Lycra, unending mirrored walls, sweat and aches. These days, gyms can be forbidding places – full of well built men admiring themselves. For others, it's a place to work out, watch your muscles grow and release the stress of the day. I have had phases in my life when I have just loved going to the gym. And others when it seemed the worst place on earth.

Exercise doesn't have to mean going to the gym. Exercise is about moving our bodies. We were meant to move – to hunt our prey, built our homes, wash our clothes, dance in triumph or worship of our gods. Our lives these days are so mechanised that we don't need to do any of these things. We can drive to work, put our clothes in the washing machine, and pull our dinner out of the microwave. As for dancing - we're usually too exhausted.

Our bodies are meant to move. Many of us have jobs that entail remaining seated for ten hours a day. We were never evolved to cope with that and bad backs often result from our endless sitting. Our sedentary world means that we need to build activity into our lives again, and this can seem artificial.

There are many benefits to exercise. As we age we lose muscle mass. And muscle is the main burner of calories in our bodies. So as we age, effectively we need fewer and fewer calories. If we can stay active, and retain some of that muscle mass, it will allow us to burn more energy which makes it easier to regulate our weigh at a healthy level. Exercise also reduces stress and helps eliminate negative chemicals, hormones and by-products from our bodies. It enhances mood and increases our immune system. It can even give you natural high.

Despite all of these benefits, many of us still see exercise as punishment. So how do we get exercise back into our lives?

Perhaps the secret is enjoyment. Our life span is limited, so lets enjoy it as much as possible. Let's find ways of being active that are pleasant, not that we have to endure.

Try to work out what you enjoy. Is it dancing to the latest hits? Or walking through a peaceful wood? Running beside the ocean? Or maybe you like the peaceful solitude of swimming laps? Or the camaraderie of team sports?

One way of rediscovering what you enjoy doing with your body is to think back to your childhood and what you enjoyed then. Did you learn ballet or tap? There are lots of classes for adults. You may feel that you could only venture into such a class once you are slim. Once you have unearthed those things that give you pleasure, build those activities into your daily life.

I enjoy dancing, walking, and running. Team sports were not my thing. I was useless at hitting any moving objects. How I hated being the last one to be picked. And then, once picked, having to humiliate myself on the field in front of everyone as I missed the ball or let my team down. Thankfully I never have to do that again.

I spent a few years trying a variety of different activities. Eventually I found which ones really suited me, which ones I enjoyed and looked forward to. For me, I discovered that if there was music going, I liked it a lot. If there weren't moving objects, I liked it even more. Once I'd identified what was fun for me, then exercise was no longer a chore.

Physical activity can help with some of those things that we often turn to food for. If you're feeling glum and low, a walk in the fresh air has been shown to be the best way to elevate mood. If you're lonely, a dance class will surround you with music and people, even if it feels hard to take the first step and get there. If you're angry and frustrated with life, one of my friends cleans the house vigorously - an activity that not only burns calories, but accomplishes a number of chores.

Try some new activities- ones that really appeal. It might be dancing round your living room to your favourite CD. Or taking up tennis again. Try going walking with a friend, or strolling out to dinner rather than driving. It can be rather nice to amble back from a dinner, hand-in-hand with your partner, chatting about the evening, and digesting the food. You might find that a 30 minute walk flies by.

If nothing else, walk round the block while you're on the phone talking. It might work against you to eat while distracted, but you can use the same logic here, and get some exercise while you're doing something else. You may not even notice it and just like the mindless snacking, your body will still respond to it, even if you don't register it.

ACTION

Remember back to when you were a child and write down the games that you used to play. Were there things that you enjoyed doing ?

Think about things you like doing physically now and write them down. It could be anything from going for a walk, to dancing in your bedroom to music, to ju jitsu or gardening.

Try to work out what it is you like about it - is it the music, or the solitude, or the team?

Use this to see whether there is something physically active that you would enjoy once a week or more.

I blame my metabolism

Metabolism is the rate at which we burn energy. Our energy comes from food, which we burn using oxygen (from our breathing). A higher or faster metabolism needs more food or fuel to keep it going.

I'd like my metabolism to be as high as possible – that way I can eat more dessert....

Many overweight individuals blame their metabolism for their weight. However, studies have shown that larger (and fatter) people have higher metabolisms, as their bodies are striving to burn up the food, and striving to move that larger person around (which takes more energy than moving a smaller person). Only in very rare cases is metabolism to blame

Generally, the person is just eating too much. I know - disappointing, hey?

There is a myth that dieting causes your metabolism to slow down. There is no evidence that dieting per se does this. Your metabolism may slow when you diet, but not because your body is trying to conserve fuel. Instead, it's because your body is burning muscle (not fat, as you'd like) to feed itself and less muscle means a slower metabolism.

So how do you go about protecting your muscle while you lose fat? The easiest way is through lifting heavy weight. Your body needs muscle to lift things, and if you are regularly using your muscles, your body won't turn to them for fuel. It will rely (reluctantly) on its fat stores.

This means that weight lifting can really assist all of us in losing weight.

For some strange reason, women think this will make them bulky. Unless you take steroids you will struggle to build muscle - let alone get bulky. We lack a number of male hormones that make it easy to build muscle. But this isn't a reason not to try. We can still build muscle that will keep us strong AND boost our metabolism.

In fact, if you lift weights, only for 20 minutes, your metabolism will remain elevated for up to two days afterwards, as your body uses calories to build the muscle it thinks it needs (as it is expecting this level of activity to continue).

The biggest muscles burn the most calories, and these are the ones in our legs and bottom. Trying to make these as big as possible, through exercising them in a gym, will yield results in terms of weight loss. For women, who are often trying to make these areas smaller, this doesn't make sense initially. But muscle is about a quarter of the size of fat: a kilo of muscle will take up a lot less room, and will burn more calories. As an added bonus, it also looks better.

Muscles in the upper body may be smaller, but they are still important for posture and strength and they still boost our metabolism.

Activities and exercise that build and maintain muscle are some of the best things we can do to maintain a healthy weight, keep ourselves active into old age. There are lots of health benefits too, like strong bones (weight bearing exercise is the best prevention against osteoporosis), a boost to the immune system and even improvements to our skin and complexion.

Some foods have been shown to elevate metabolism. These include:
Cinnamon

Chillies

Coffee

However, the effect on the metabolism is minimal - we are talking a few calories only, so loading up on these isn't the answer.

Getting cold or being in a cool room also forces your metabolism to kick in to keep you warm. The very act of eating causes your metabolism to fire up. But, sadly, not by enough to make a real difference. Increasing muscle mass is the surest way to boost the rate at which we burn energy.

Even so, increasing your metabolism won't give you carte blanche to plough into a massive tub of ice cream without putting on weight. But regular weight training and an increased amount of muscle in your body will definitely give you more leeway.

Our metabolisms aren't to blame for our health issues, but we can keep them revved up by maintaining our muscle mass. Otherwise, any variance in metabolism isn't large enough to make a difference.

ACTION

If you want to increase your metabolism, try to build more muscle. This is easiest at the gym with weights, but can also be achieved through anything that taxes your body - even lifting heavy bags of shopping will keep you strong.

Because I'm too damn busy

Stephanie works in a hospital. Her days are frantic - a literal matter of life and death. Her shifts are long and arduous and when she gets home she has two small children that she has to to feed, bathe, get to bed, play with and be mother to. Her husband? I guess he gets a look in, now and then...

She is would like to lose a little weight but has no time to prepare food, so finds herself ravenous in the middle of her shift and grabs something from the vending machine. Then guilt assails her. She, of all people, working in medicine, knows how she should be eating. Pushing that thought aside, she carries on with her crazy schedule.

When she gets home, she feeds the kids, intending to eat later with her husband. Somehow, she ends up eating with them, as she's starving. Then she cooks another meal, her husband gets home, and she eats again with him. She barely has a moment to herself, let alone a moment to think about what she's eating.

Our lives are so busy, that this is true for many of us. Many parents find themselves eating with the children as well as later. This is partly because we are hungry and exhausted by this stage, and need some sustenance to keep us going. It's also because socially it is quite awkward to sit with others while they eat and not eat yourself.

It might seem tricky, but it's worth trying to carve out fifteen minutes a day, either to have a rest (rather than a snack) as mentioned earlier, or to plan out our eating for the week. It's hard when surrounded by the demands of a job and children and a household and a spouse or partner. Sometimes it comes down to a question of what is the priority in your life. It is quite legitimate to put weight loss or how you eat much lower on the list now and then. It is also legitimate to put a little time aside to look after yourself so that you can better look after others.

I saw it on Instagram!

"I examine the 'before' photo closely. It could be me. Bra digging into the shoulders, flesh bulging around the straps. The face is full - not quite a double chin, but nearly. I usually tell yourself it's a bad angle when I see photos of myself like that. Her arms are meaty, her top loose. Mine too - it covers the roll that oozes over my waistband, a doughy roll that even my stretch jeans can't contain.

"Then the 'after' photo. Could that also be me, one day? Her abdomen is lean and lightly muscled. She isn't tall - not a model then. Her legs look great - slim and toned. Her gaze is coolly confident. None of the shame and embarrassment that I usually feel about myself.

"I scroll through the photos of her food. It looks generous and colourful. My mouth waters. Eggs, their yolks yellow and luscious, drip onto green avocado. There is even toast. Toast! The porridge has chocolate and peanut butter. I moisten my lips. I could do that, no problem. I buy the book.

"I start with the chocolate porridge. The oat bran turns grey in the cooking water and boiling it for a few minutes, it has the consistency and colour of dirty dishwater. The chocolate protein powder, too, has a faint grey hue, and immediately congeals into large lumps. I spoon it into a bowl. The serving looks small, apologetic almost. I'd been salivating over chocolate peanut butter porridge. The peanut butter on top so meagre that I can barely notice it. It doesn't taste as I'd hoped. The flavour reminds me of soggy cardboard except that the protein powder has acquired a consistency remarkably similar to grit. I can't taste either chocolate or peanuts. Maybe I should slap a larger tablespoon of the latter on top. Surely it wouldn't hurt?

"Somehow none of the recipes, when I make them, look like the pictures. The salad that looks so delicious in the photos is only a collection of raw cabbage and leaves. There is no dressing or mayonnaise. I chew on it, like a cow ruminating on the cud. The cabbage sticks in my teeth. I used to like coleslaw. I hate cabbage, I think. An hour later, I'm hungry.

"By the time I get home, my boss has been a nightmare and my workload has doubled. That night I don't want the quinoa salad. I want ice cream. A large serve of creamy ice cream, eaten straight from the tub in front of the television. Just tonight, I say, just tonight and then tomorrow, back onto the porridge.

"A week later the book lies unopened on the shelf. My jeans are a little tighter. I turn away from my reflection. I'll never look like the after photo. I'm not good enough. I'm weak. I couldn't even stick it out for a day. What's the point in even trying?

"I may as well have those chips. The takeaway is only a short drive away. After the disappointment you need some comfort. And a large bowl of hot chips is the best comfort I can think of. I turn off Instagram and get into the car.

"I'll never be the 'after' girl."

Are you waiting for your own Cinderella or Instagram story? Do you sometimes feel like you are dressed in rags, or cloaked in extra pounds, your beauty unnoticed? Are you waiting for your fairy godmother to clothe you in radiance so that you can, at long last, walk into the room, and have everyone see you for what you are, everyone gasp at your beauty, everyone want to know you?

Are you waiting to climb out of the ashes, and step into a golden carriage? Or at the very least, at BMW...?

Perhaps the latest health fad or gimmick is the wand that will wave the transformation? The magic dust that will sprinkle over your life, dissolving the roll around the middle, and smoothing out the other wrinkles in your existence.

There is a fairy godmother who can do this. But that fairy godmother is you. You have to do it for yourself. And it's going to take rather longer than the wave of a wand. But it can happen.

And you can make it.

The Instagram feeds and diet blogs of today promise even more immediate dreams and results than the eating plans in magazines. The problem is that we can't see or taste the reality. The photos of the food may look beautiful, but there is nothing about how they taste. It's easy to make a gorgeous image of colourful ingredients - much harder to make it delicious. We know now that we 'eat with our eyes', and Instagram fools us into thinking that because an image of a recipe looks pretty, then it will taste the same. Sadly, when the ingredients are poor imitations of food, or lacking fat or carbohydrate, it is unlikely.

Likewise the images of the bodies. Some backlash has begun and even the Instastars are admitting that their lives and figures aren't as perfect as they might have led us to believe. One or two have suffered depression and anxiety due to the discrepancy between what they are depicting and their reality. An Australian teenager with more than half a million followers on Instagram has quit it, describing it as 'contrived perfection made to get attention'.

If you feel yourself sucked into the vortex of perfect bodies and perfect eating, cling onto something real for support.

ACTION

Try to remember that social media is not real life. If you feel yourself being attracted to what is displayed on it, spend more time with real people, to get a balanced view of how we each struggle with our lives our bodies and our relationships.

IN CLOSING

"We are all different, in lifestyle, genetics and psychology. What is effective, healthy and realistic for one, might be the opposite for someone else. Often this is hard for people writing diet books to grasp."

Anthony Warner, aka 'The Angry Chef'

We've covered a lot of ground in this book.

We began by looking at the way we set ourselves up to fail, for which the diet industry must take a large portion of the blame. We aren't helped by food manufacturers. While the advent of processed and packaged foods frees us all up from having to spend time in the kitchen, over recent years this seems to be at the expense of our health, or at least our ability to eat in a measured way. These processing of foods messes with our body chemistry and with the neurochemistry in our brains to make us overeat.

"My biggest concern with losing weight rapidly is the affect it has on someone's mental wellbeing," says Dr Frankie Phillips, registered dietitian and nutritionist and spokesperson for the British Dietetic Association. "Crash diets often leave people feeling demoralised when they start to regain weight so quickly."

A review published by Yale University's Department of Psychology acknowledged the correlation between yo-yo dieting (or weight cycling) and mental health issues. "Weight cycling appears linked to increased psychopathology, lower life satisfaction, more disturbed eating in general and perhaps increased risk for binge eating," it says.

More and more research is pointing to the damage done by dieting and restricted eating. No wonder we cheat.

Finally we have explored ways that we might break free of 'cheating' while we eat, and sabotaging ourselves. There is a vast amount and array of information in this area, and I have attempted to present the highlights of my research in a digestible manner.

A researcher (Timmerman) recently suggested a term to describe the psychological state of eating less than one wants: perceived deprivation. She has shown that, among obese women who regularly engaged in binge eating, caloric intake on the days prior to their highest calorie binge days did not reflect low calorie dieting. They were eating, on average 2200 calories, but they own estimates. And because we know individuals substantially under-report their caloric intake, this figure is probably an underestimate of the truth. Timmerman has shown that scores on this measure of perceived deprivation, which were collected daily for 14 days, did not correlate with actual caloric intake on the same day, indicating that perceived deprivation did not stem from actual caloric deprivation.

These results are consistent with the arguments that many individuals may experience a sense of deprivation not because they are eating less than they need but because they are eating less than they want. Deprivation isn't real - our bodies aren't calorie-deprived, we just feel that we are because we aren't eating what we want to eat.

Recent studies on an animal model of binge eating have produced results consistent with this viewpoint. In fact, I had a discussion with the nutritionist from one of Australia's top zoos, and her experience with animals is similar. I marvel that they suffer the way we do. Remove their favourite treats and the animals exhibit signs of depression and low mood.

What is clear, and proven by science is that the motivation to eat more than we need is every bit as real, and, perhaps, every bit as powerful, as the motivation to eat when truly energy deprived. This is why dieting is so dangerous. The feeling of deprivation emerges almost immediately. The power of eating what you want when you feel like it, attuned to your internal cues, allow you to avoid this sense of poverty, of wanting, of being deprived.

In summary, it helps if you keep your blood sugar reasonably stable. To do this, eat plenty of protein, ideally with every meal, don't eat too much sugar or high glycemic foods (or artificial sweeteners), and try not to drip feed food into your system. Give it a break now and then. Wait for hunger - this is your body communicating with you, and besides, it is the best seasoning.

Allow yourself to eat your favourite foods. Allow yourself to enjoy your meals: the sense of deprivation is the enemy of weight management. Work out what it takes for you to feel satisfied, and have that, or do that.

Don't listen to other people, whether it's your mother, the latest diet book or your new boyfriend. Only you can know what's best for you. Be brave and listen to your body and preferences. Sleep when you're tired, rest when you need to and look after yourself. You are more precious than you know.

Keep reading in the area. Scientists are making advances all the time.

Armed with this knowledge, I hope that we all feel empowered to make the decisions that are right for us. this is going to be different for everyone, as we all have different genetic codes, different backgrounds and family traditions, and different psychology. Sadly, this has meant that there is not one set of rules that will fix this for everyone. It means that we each have to find our own way.

I hope that this books helps you find your way, a way that is sustainable and enjoyable for you, a way that means you celebrate your life, enjoy your food, and fully inhabit the marvellous body that you were born in.

Give yourself permission. To eat, to not eat. To choose. To find your way, the way that works for you.

A summary of techniques and ideas.

The Basics
- Give up all diets and restrictive eating plans
- There is no need to cut out any major food groups
- Discover what you enjoy eating and what makes you feel good
- Wait until you're hungry before you eat
- Work out what you'd like to eat
- Eat what you're hungry for, what you really want
- Make time to enjoy it and focus on it
- Eat until you are satisfied and then stop

Help your body work with you
- Rest when you're tired
- Get enough sleep
- Keep blood sugar level by
- eating regular protein
- Not eating too many sugary or high carbohydrate foods
- Not eating too often - give your stomach time to rest
- Eat a balanced and varied diet that includes protein, fats and carbs
- Eat fruit and vegetables to help your microbiome

Deal with Addictive Foods and Behaviours
- Know that processed foods are designed to be addictive and choose how you want to deal with that
- Accept that sometimes one taste will make you want more than you might choose to eat, and decide whether you really want that taste
- Make it easier to break habits, or stop your brain over-riding your resolution, by changing what foods you keep at home, or other triggering events

Get your brain in gear

- Recognise that if you're 'cheating' then some part of you isn't signed up to what you're doing
- If you've failed at dieting, let go of the belief that it was you at fault. It's always the diet that's unreasonable
- If the desire to eat rises from external cues, whether cakes at work, walking past a bakery or seeing an advert for food, check in with yourself and ask if you really want it. Promise yourself that you can have it when you do.
- Plan how you're going to approach social events and meals out
- Recognise that beliefs aren't set in stone: you can change them

When it all goes wrong

- If you eat more than you're comfortable with, recognise that as something we all do on occasion
- If you've eaten too much, try to be kinder to yourself than usual
- Work out what else is going on that is making you need to lean on food
- Get professional help if things are going seriously pear-shaped

The Icing on the Cake

- Imagine eating what you're craving, for at least thirty times
- Promise yourself unlimited amounts of your forbidden or danger foods tomorrow and see how much you want it today
- Blindfold yourself when eating
- Love your thighs
- Be kind to yourself
- And finally: ignore all my rules and make your own.

CITATIONS, REFERENCES AND SOURCES

Misattribution of reasons why we do things

Dutton, D.G.; Aaron, A. P. (1974). "Some evidence for heightened sexual attraction under conditions of high anxiety". Journal of Personality and Social Psychology. 30 (4): 510–517

Minnesota Starvation Experiment

Keys, A., Brozek, J., Henshel, A., Mickelson, O., & Taylor, H.L. (1950). The biology of human starvation, (Vols. 1–2). Minneapolis, MN: University of Minnesota Press.

Tucker, T. (2007). The great starvation experiment: Ancel Keys and the men who starved for science. Minneapolis, MN: University of Minnesota Press.

Dieting increases likelihood of eating disorder for 18 times.

Patton G C, Selzer R, Coffey C, Carlin J B, Wolfe R. Onset of adolescent eating disorders: population based cohort study over 3 years BMJ 1999; 318 :765

Diets fail and Dieters regain weight

Mann, T., Tomiyama, A. J., Westling, E., Lew, A.-M., Samuels, B., & Chatman, J. (2007). Medicare's search for effective obesity treatments: Diets are not the answer. American Psychologist, 62(3), 220-233.

Wolfgang Stroebe, Wendy Mensink, Henk Aarts, Henk Schut, Arie W. Kruglanskib. Why dieters fail: Testing the goal conflict model of eating. Journal of Experimental Social Psychology, Vol 44, Issue 1, January 2008, Pages 26-36

K H Pietiläinen, S E Saarni, J Kaprio & A Rissanen. Does dieting make you fat? A twin study. International Journal of Obesity (2012) 36, pages 456–464

Paul S. MacLean, Audrey Bergouignan, Marc-Andre Cornier, and Matthew R. Jackman. Biology's response to dieting: the impetus for weight regain. American Journal of Physiology Regulatory Integrative and Comparative Physiology Vol 301, No 3: R581–R600, 2011.

Michael R.Lowe, Rachel A. Annunziatoa, Jessica Tuttman Markowitz, Elizabeth Didie, Dara L. Bellace, Lynn Riddell, Caralynn Maille, Shortie McKinney, Eric Stice. Multiple types of dieting prospectively predict weight gain during the freshman year of college. Appetite, Vol 47, Issue 1, July 2006, Pages 83-90

Palascha, A., van Kleef, E., & van Trijp, H. C. (2015). How does thinking in Black and White terms relate to eating behavior and weight regain?. Journal of health psychology, 20(5), 638-648.

Byrne, S. M., Cooper, Z., & Fairburn, C. G. (2004). Psychological predictors of weight regain in obesity. Behaviour research and therapy, 42(11), 1341-1356.

Sairanen, E., Lappalainen, R., Lapveteläinen, A., Tolvanen, A., & Karhunen, L. (2014). Flexibility in weight management. Eating behaviors, 15(2), 218-224.

Meule, A., Westenhöfer, J., & Kübler, A. (2011). Food cravings mediate the relationship between rigid, but not flexible control of eating behavior and dieting success. Appetite, 57(3), 582-584.

Smith, C. F., Williamson, D. A., Bray, G. A., & Ryan, D. H. (1999). Flexible vs. Rigid dieting strategies: relationship with adverse behavioral outcomes. Appetite, 32(3), 295-305.

Efficacy of Protein

Veldhorst, Westerterp, van Vught, Westerterp-Plantenga. Presence or absence of carbohydrates and the proportion of fat in a high-protein diet affect appetite suppression but not energy expenditure in normal-weight human subjects fed in energy balance. British Journal of Nutrition. 2010 Nov;104(9):1395-405

Westerterp-Plantenga MS, Lejeune MP. Protein intake and body-weight regulation. Appetite. 2005 Oct;45(2):187-90.

D M Dreon, B Frey-Hewitt, N Ellsworth, P T Williams, R B Terry, and P D Wood. Dietary fat:carbohydrate ratio and obesity in middle-aged men. American Journal Clinical Nutrition, June 1988, vol. 47 no. 6, 995-1000

Dangers of fasting

David S. Weigle P. Barton Duell William E. Connor Robert A. Steiner Michael R. Soules Joseph L. Kuijper. Effect of Fasting, Refeeding, and Dietary Fat Restriction on Plasma Leptin Levels. The Journal of Clinical Endocrinology & Metabolism, Volume 82, Issue 2, 1 February 1997, Pages 561–565

Pietiläinen KH et al. Inaccuracies in food and physical activity diaries of obese subjects: complementary evidence from doubly labeled water and co-twin assessments. International Journal of Obesity (London). 2010 Mar; 34(3):437-45.

Lack of sleep

Erin C. Hanlon, Esra Tasali, Rachel Leproult, Kara L. Stuhr, BS Elizabeth Doncheck, Harriet de Wit, Cecilia J. Hillard, Eve Van Cauter. Sleep Restriction Enhances the Daily Rhythm of Circulating Levels of Endocannabinoid 2-Arachidonoylglycerol. Sleep, Volume 39, Issue 3, 1 March 2016, Pages 653–664,

Stevia and artificial sweeteners

P.B.Jeppesen et al. Stevioside acts directly on pancreatic β cells to secrete insulin: Actions independent of cyclic adenosine monophosphate and adenosine triphosphate—sensitivie K+-channel activity. Metabolism, Vol 49, Issue 2, Feb 2000, Pages 208-214

Michael GTordoff Annette MAlleva. Oral stimulation with

aspartame increases hunger. Physiology & Behavior, Vol 47, Issue 3, March 1990, Pages 555-559

Qing Yang. Gain weight by "going diet?" Artificial sweeteners and the neurobiology of sugar cravings. Yale Journal of Biology and Medicine. 2010 Jun; 83(2): 101–108.

Sugar

Ferris Jabr. How Sugar and Fat Trick the Brain into Wanting More Food: Junk foods can muddle the brain's satiety-control mechanism, sending our appetites into hyperdrive. Scientific American, January 1, 2016

Lenoir M, Serre F, Cantin L, Ahmed SH (2007) Intense Sweetness Surpasses Cocaine Reward. PLoS ONE 2(8): e698.

Arthur N. Westover, Lauren B. Marangell. A cross-national relationship between sugar consumption and major depression? Depression and Anxiety, Vol 16, Issue 3, 2002, Pages 118–120.

Hedonic Hunger

Michael R.Lowe and Meghan L. Butryn. Hedonic hunger: A new dimension of appetite? Physiology & Behavior, Vol 91, Iss 4, 24 July 2007, Pages 432-439

Michael R. Lowe, Allen S. Levine. Eating Motives and the Controversy over Dieting: Eating Less Than Needed versus Less Than Wanted. Obesity, Vol 13, Issue 5, May 2005, Pages 797–806

Gluten-free

B. Zanini et al. Randomised clinical study: gluten challenge induces symptom recurrence in only a minority of patients who meet clinical criteria for non-coeliac gluten sensitivity. Alimentary Pharmacology and Therapeutics. Volume 42, Issue 8, October 2015, Pages 968–976

Biesiekierski JR, Peters SL, Newnham ED, Rosella O, Muir JG,

Gibson PR. No effects of gluten in patients with self-reported non-celiac gluten sensitivity after dietary reduction of fermentable, poorly absorbed, short-chain carbohydrates. Gastroenterology. 2013 Aug; 145(2):3 20-8

Visual stimulation, priming

Charles Spence, Katsunori Okajima, Adrian David Cheok, Olivia Petit, Charles Michel. Eating with our eyes: From visual hunger to digital satiation. Brain and Cognition, Volume 110, December 2016, Pages 53-63

Stice, E., Spoor, S., Bohon, C., Veldhuizen, M. G., & Small, D. M. (2008). Relation of reward from food intake and anticipated food intake to obesity: A functional magnetic resonance imaging study. Journal of Abnormal Psychology, 117(4), 924-935.

Harris, J. L., Bargh, J. A., & Brownell, K. D. (2009). Priming effects of television food advertising on eating behavior. Health Psychology, 28(4), 404-413.

Carol E.Cornell, Judith Rodin, Harvey Weingarten. Stimulus-induced eating when satiated. Physiology & Behavior, Volume 45, Issue 4, April 1989, Pages 695-704

Imagining eating

Carey K. Morewedge, Young Eun Huh, Joachim Vosgerau. Thought for Food: Imagined Consumption Reduces Actual Consumption. Science 10 Dec 2010: Vol. 330, Issue 6010, pp. 1530-1533

Jane Ogden, Jane Wardle. Cognitive restraint and sensitivity to cues for hunger and satiety. Physiology & Behavior, Volume 47, Issue 3, March 1990, Pages 477-481

Chocolate

Bruinsma K, Taren D L. Chocolate: Food or Drug? Journal of

the American Dietetic Association, Vol 99, Issue 10, October 1999, Pages 1249-1256

Andrea L. Tranquilli et all. Female fetuses are more reactive when mother eats chocolate. The Journal of Maternal-Fetal & Neonatal Medicine, Vol 27, 2014 - Issue 1, pages 72-74.

Losing weight

Ruben Meerman, and Andrew J Brown. When somebody loses weight, where does the fat go? British Medical Journal 2014;349:g7257

Fatemeh Azizi Soeliman and Leila Azadbakht. Weight loss maintenance: A review on dietary related strategies. Journal of Research in Medical Sciences. 2014 Mar; 19(3): 268–275.

Alajmi, N et al. Appetite and Energy Intake Responses to Acute Energy Deficits in Females versus Males. Medicine & Science in Sports & Exercise: March 2016 - Volume 48 - Issue 3 - p 412–420

Processed food

Anthony Sclafani and Deleri Springer. Dietary obesity in adult rats: Similarities to hypothalamic and human obesity syndromes. Physiology & Behavior, Volume 17, Issue 3, September 1976, Pages 461-471

Jacques Peretti. Why our food is making us fat. The Guardian, June 11, 2012.

Madison Park. Twinkie diet helps nutrition professor lose 27 pounds. CNN, Nov 8 2010.

Gut

Anthony Sclafani. Gut–brain nutrient signaling. Appetition vs. satiation. Appetite, Volume 71, 1 December 2013, Pages 454-458

Vic Norrisa, Franck Molinab and Andrew T. Gewirtz. Hypothesis: Bacteria Control Host Appetites. Journal of

Bacteriology. February 2013 vol. 195 no. 3 pages 411-416

Flint, Harry J. Obesity and the Gut Microbiota. Journal of Clinical Gastroenterology: Nov/Dec 2011, Vol 45, Issue - p S128–S132

Sonnenburg, J and Sonnenburg E. Gut Feelings–the "Second Brain" in Our Gastrointestinal Systems. Scientific American. May 2015.

Metabolism

Petra Stiegler, Adam Cunliffe. The Role of Diet and Exercise for the Maintenance of Fat-Free Mass and Resting Metabolic Rate During Weight Loss. Sports Medicine, March 2006, Volume 36, Issue 3, pp 239–262

Stress

Ward, A., & Mann, T. (2000). Don't mind if I do: Disinhibited eating under cognitive load. Journal of Personality and Social Psychology, 78(4), 753-763.

Femke Rutters, Arie G. Nieuwenhuizen, Sofie G.T. Lemmens, Jurriaan M. Born, Margriet S. Westerterp-Planten. Acute Stress-related Changes in Eating in the Absence of Hunger. Obesity, Vol 17, Issue 1, Jan 2009, Pages 72–77

Social pressures

Duncker, K. (1938). Experimental modification of children's food preferences through social suggestion. The Journal of Abnormal and Social Psychology, 33(4), 489-507.

Peter J Rogers, Hendrik J Smit. Food Craving and Food "Addiction": A Critical Review of the Evidence From a Biopsychosocial Perspective. Pharmacology Biochemistry and Behavior, Volume 66, Issue 1, May 2000, Pages 3-14

Marshmallow test

Mischel, W., Ebbesen, E. B., & Raskoff Zeiss, A. (1972). Cognitive and attentional mechanisms in delay of gratification. Journal of Personality and Social Psychology, 21(2), 204-218.

Deprivation

Gayle M. Timmerman, Elizabeth K. Gregg. Dieting, Perceived Deprivation, and Preoccupation with Food. Western Journal of Nursing Research. Vol 25, Issue 4, 2003

Books:

Michael Pollan: In Defence of Food. Penguin 2008.

Gary Taubes: Why we get fat. Anchor Books 2010.

Dr Rick Kausman: If not dieting, then what? Allen & Unwin 1998.

Giulia Enders: Gut. Scribe 2014.

Genuine Roth: Breaking Free from Compulsive Eating. Penguin 1996.

Susie Orbach: Fat is a Feminist Issue. Hamlyn 1984.

E Tribole and E Resch: Intuitive Eating. Griffin 1995.

ABOUT THE AUTHOR

Clare Taylor has an honours degree in Psychology. She has worked in marketing for a number of the world's large food manufacturers.

She now works as a diet coach, mentoring those who feel trapped by their weight and out of control of their eating. She encourages her clients to let go of diets and learn a new way, a way of working with their bodies and natural appetite to maintain a healthy weight while still enjoying a wide variety of food.

She has lived in the UK, South Africa and Australia.

Currently, she calls Sydney home.

Find her, along with more great tips at: dietcoach.blog